RECIPES FOR

Candida Albicans

RECIPES FOR HEALTH

Candida Albicans

Over 100 yeast-free and sugar-free recipes

SHIRLEY TRICKETT

Thorsons
An Imprint of HarperCollinsPublishers

Thorsons
An Imprint of HarperCollins*Publishers*
77–85 Fulham Palace Road,
Hammersmith, London W6 8JB
1160 Battery Sreet
San Francisco, California 94111–1213

Published by Thorsons 1995
3 5 7 9 10 8 6 4 2

A catalogue record for this book
is available from the British Library

ISBN 0 7225 2967 8

Printed and bound in Great Britain by
Caledonian International Book Manufacturing Ltd, Glasgow

Contents

Introduction

THE DANGER OF DIY DIAGNOSIS

I MUST STRESS that no matter how closely you can identify your symptoms with those mentioned in this book, you **must** see your doctor before embarking on self help programmes, because the same symptoms can arise in other conditions. Also you will see that some drugs are implicated in causing the candida problem. Do not cut down or discontinue these or any other prescribed drugs without the approval of your doctor. If you are diabetic or have been given a diet chart from your doctor for any reason check with him/her before you make any changes.

There is increasing evidence to show that people are succumbing to more fungal infections than ever before. However, the good news is that the symptoms of Candida Albicans (thrush) and other yeasts (fungus) respond very well to diet, natural anti-candida treatment and general health care. You **can** feel fit again even if your symptoms are very severe.

PHYSICAL PROBLEMS

Skin conditions: cracks at the corners of the mouth, spots under the skin, itching scaly rashes often on the face in women and around the genitals in men, athlete's foot

Nail-bed infections

Ear, nose and throat infections, mouth ulcers

Asthma

Conjunctivitis

Sinusitis

Chronic cystitis

Vaginal and oral thrush

Hormonal imbalance: water retention, PMT, period pain

Both underweight and overweight: inability to lose weight on a low calorie diet

Digestive disturbances such as nausea, bloating, altered bowel habits, inflammation of the whole of the digestive tract from the mouth to the anus, food cravings, food intolerance

Allergies

Muscle and joint pains.

WHEN CANDIDA TAKES OVER

Candida normally lives in the bowel from infancy and providing there are enough good bacteria available to keep it under control all is well. If, however, the immune system is not working well either because of illness,

Candida Albicans

drugs, poor diet or stress, the delicate ecological balance in the gut is destroyed and the fungus can take over. When this happens the bowel becomes an overactive fermentation tank; a great deal of gas is formed causing abdominal bloating and digestive disturbances. Part of the reason for this is that the fungus blocks the sites where enzymes – chemicals necessary for the breaking down of the food we eat – are produced. Candida overgrowth also inhibits the production of vitamins normally made in the bowel. This is why a person on an adequate diet can show signs of vitamin deficiency.

CHRONIC OR SYSTEMIC CANDIDIASIS

When there is a proliferation of candida the yeast cell can change from its simple form (which looks like a fried egg) to its complicated mycelial form (which looks like a battered fried egg with roots). These roots can penetrate the bowel wall allowing not only the toxins (which include alcohol) made by the candida to escape into the circulation, but also gives the organism a chance to infect other sites in the body. This gives rise to the condition known as Systemic Candidiasis, an illness which often defies diagnosis. The reason for this is, because of the wide range of physical and psychiatric symptoms the patient is often thought to be a hypochondriac. Doctors who are not trained in Clinical Nutrition usually only expect to see systemic candidiasis arising as a complication in severely debilitated patients with life-threatening

diseases, and even if they do suspect some of your symptoms are caused by a fungal overgrowth in the bowel,
they are unlikely to give the prolonged antifungal
therapy needed or give dietary advice. This is why so
many people turn to self-help methods.

PSYCHOLOGICAL SYMPTOMS

When the toxins escape from the bowel, which instead of
being a sealed unit is now like a leaking hosepipe, they
can travel to the brain and cause:

- Headaches
- Irritability
- Confusion
- Mood swings
- Agitation
- Anxiety
- Depression

Many candida sufferers who have had symptoms for
years, 'the thick file patients', respond very well to the
self-help programme described and find their self-esteem
again after years of being labelled neurotic. Their intui-
tive knowledge of their bodies convinces them that their
symptoms have a physical basis.

MEDICAL AWARENESS OF THE CANDIDA PROBLEM

In general this is poor, except for doctors trained in Clinical Nutrition. In America, the pioneering work of doctors O C Truss and William Crook has done a lot to educate both the profession and the public, but as with anything else considered new in medicine it takes a long time to filter through and be generally accepted.

WHY IS THERE AN INCREASE IN FUNGAL INFECTIONS?

The way we live in the twentieth century is slowly weakening the human immune system and the body is no longer able to cope with organisms such as the parasitic yeast candida albicans. The damage is being done by:

Junk foods
Rise in consumption of sugar
The stress of modern life
Ever-increasing consumption of alcohol
Street drugs
Environmental pollutants
The use of more drugs prescribed than ever before in history, many of which actively encourage fungal growth and depress the immune system. They include:
    The pill
    Antibiotics

Steroids
Tranquillisers and sleeping pills
Ulcer drugs

Some of the medicines involved in causing the candida problem are undoubtedly vital in life-threatening illnesses, but the injudicious use of them can also be life-threatening, or at the very least can cause chronic minor problems that keep people permanently below par.

GIVING THE CANDIDA
A HARD TIME

If your symptoms are severe it is advisable to see your physician or a doctor who specializes in clinical nutrition. Whilst a hospital dietician will probably have very little knowledge of a diet designed to control candida, there are alternative practitioners such as naturopaths, homœopaths and nutrition counsellors (see pages 140–4) who have a wealth of information and experience. There are also candida self-help counselling lines (see pages 140–4).

Fortunately, candida responds well to self-help methods. The approach is safe and effective although it may take many months. The treatment consists not only of killing the candida with non-drug, anti-fungal agents, such as garlic or substances from the coconut or castor bean oil, but also by transforming the habitat of the candida from Shangri La to the Sahara desert. To achieve this, the bowel is kept as clean as possible and re-colonized with good

Candida Albicans

bacteria such as *Lactobacillus acidophilus* which is available in live yogurt or in some health supplements. In addition, olive oil and yeast-free minerals and vitamins are taken to strengthen the immune system. This further discourages candida growth; as does a healthy diet devoid of sugar, refined carbohydrate, yeast-containing foods, and all fermented products. When fresh air, sunlight, adequate rest and exercise are added, this rogue yeast has to retreat with its tails between its legs.

WHAT THIS BOOK HAS TO OFFER

This book describes eating plans for moderate symptoms and a stricter diet for those who want to kill off the candida more quickly. The reasons why certain foods should be avoided are explained. It also gives a cleansing, soothing seven-day plan for people who have inflammation of the digestive system. This one is also helpful for weight reduction.

WHICH DIET FOR YOU?

It would be impossible to give a specific eating plan which would suit everyone as there are so many factors to consider; the severity of your symptoms, your weight, the state of your digestive system, what, if any, food intolerances you have, your lifestyle – how much time you have to prepare food, your financial situation, and how drastic changes in your diet are going to affect your state of mind – are you going to feel miserable and deprived? The answer would seem to be, keep a balance (unless you have dietary instructions from your doctor), avoid the main foods which encourage candida growth, take a natural antifungal substance, and if your symptoms don't improve seek professional guidance. Although it has to be said that diets recommended by practitioners vary a great deal. Some say eat as much complex carbohydrate, such as brown rice, as you like, others restrict this. Others encourage eating more protein, meat, fish, poultry, eggs, nuts and pulses to keep the blood sugar stable, avoiding that sinking mid-morning and mid-afternoon feeling which makes your body scream for a sugar 'fix'. It is very important to be aware of the low blood sugar/candida connection. For more on blood sugar levels read *Coping Successfully with Panic Attacks* (see Further Reading, page 139). My own observations are equally confusing. I have seen people bloom on the strict vegetarian/naturopathic approach, whilst others have failed to lose weight (perhaps because of a genetic inability to metabolize carbohydrate) and others who have had a dramatic weight loss and consequent loss of energy. I have also seen many people who do well by simply cutting out bread, sugar and the foods at the top of the banned list, increasing their intake of vegetables, salads and fruit, and taking supplements. They continue eating bacon or eggs for breakfast, meat when they want it, and by restricting their grain intake to four to six Ryvita or rice cakes daily, lose weight and their candida problems. It is going to be up to you to find the eating plan which suits you best but do give any change in diet, time. You may lose weight at first then stabilize, equally if you are overweight you might not see results for several weeks. Also be prepared in the early days to have withdrawal symptoms such as headaches, aching muscles, food cravings and low mood. They will pass after a few days. They are a sign that your body is getting rid of toxins.

STRICT DIETING

This book strives for balance, for whilst listing certain foods as forbidden for those who want to relieve severe symptoms, it also has choices for those who are over the worst and want a more relaxed approach. My experience of many people faced with a strict, unfamiliar way of eating (boiled oats or millet without sugar or salt, soya milk instead of cows' milk, plus salads and vegetables) is that unless they are motivated by feeling very unwell or have close counselling support, they simply do not keep to their diet and swing from dieting to their old eating habits, thereby delaying their progress and also becoming annoyed with themselves. There is frustration for the therapist too when they are faced with someone saying 'But I did not have time, I grabbed a sandwich and a Mars bar.'

SUPPLEMENTS

Guidance on drug and nondrug antifungal substances and supplements to boost the immune system are given in

Candida Albicans – Could Yeast Be your Problem (see Further Reading, page 138).

RECIPES

This is not a gourmet cookery book. The recipes are simple and designed to fit in with family meals. They concentrate on foods which will not encourage fungal growth – as yeast-free and sugar-free as possible and high in vegetable fibre, as well as bringing out the natural sugars in foods and slowly re-educating the palate. Some of the recipes contain small amounts of 'forbidden foods'. Don't be surprised at this – there is a great deal of difference between eating a large wedge of Cheddar and adding a sprinkling of grated cheese to give the final touch to a dish.

Most of the ingredients are available on any supermarket shelf. Those that aren't can be bought in any health food store. The reasons why certain foods, such as olive oil, are emphasized, are explained.

EQUIPMENT

Remembering the students and low income people with ill-equipped kitchens I have seen, I have tried to keep the equipment required to a minimum – a baking sheet, a decent-sized frying pan with a lid (or you can use a baking sheet), a couple of saucepans, a chopping board and a sharp vegetable knife.

FOOD SHOULD BE FUN

Food is one of the main pleasures in life so in keeping to more familiar tastes you will feel less deprived and much more willing to continue long term with healthier eating. You will have to accept that the days of eating toast or sugar-laden cereal for breakfast, a sandwich for lunch, a large evening meal and biscuits and nibbles later are over if you want to make your digestive tract an inhospitable place for the candida and regain your health. A diet should be regarded as a medicine which can correct imbalances in your body chemistry, and strengthen your immune system to cope with disease. Like any medicine it might need changing from time to time. If you are very depleted, a course of vitamins and minerals (see *Coping with Candida*, Further Reading, page 139) could accelerate your recovery. Above all *relax*. If you are going to worry about every morsel that passes your lips – will this upset me, will this make the candida grow? – then you are providing just what the candida needs. Stress is a great strain on the immune system.

FOOD INTOLERANCES

It would be difficult to provide recipes to cater for individual needs since many people with candida have food intolerances. I have tried to overcome this to a degree by giving alternatives to the main food allergens such as wheat and dairy products.

YOUR OTHER NEEDS

A healthy diet alone will not restore you to vibrant health. Your immune system also needs adequate rest, exercise, fresh air, sunshine and most of all it is vital that you get to know yourself, find out where your major stresses are coming from. Do you put the needs of others before your own? Do you rush around when you could take life at a more leisurely pace? Do you let fear dominate your life? As you clear the candida and harmful toxins from your body, it could also be the time to face habitual negative emotions, discover the lonely inner child within you, and by accepting and learning to love that child, find the peace that allows you to connect with your higher self and your purpose.

1

Choosing Ingredients

THE FRESHER foods are, the less likely they are to harbour moulds. Shop where there is a quick turnover of products and refrigerate goods as soon as possible. Ideally, candida sufferers should choose organic products but the increased cost and poor availability often do not make this an option.

VEGETABLES AND FRUIT

Pass over wilting greens and root vegetables, and courgettes, onions and peppers that are not really hard to the touch. People often reason that if the vegetables are going to be cooked it does not matter if they are not as crisp as they should be. There are two reasons why this is not so – not only do mould spores love wilting vegetables, but also ageing vegetables lose nutrients and vital energy.

Mushrooms: Unless you know you are sensitive to mushrooms there should be no reason why they cannot be included in your diet. They are low carbohydrate and do not feed candida.

Fresh fruit: This can be included after the first three weeks unless your symptoms are severe. The bloom on fruit is mould. It should therefore be peeled.

MEAT

It is better to avoid beef and pork (unless they are organic) if your symptoms are severe, since they often contain antibiotics or steroids, both of which encourage candida growth. If they are normally part of your diet and you would miss them, you could take them occasionally if you are on a maintenance diet. Lamb is a better choice.

POULTRY

Fresh, free range, corn-fed birds (unless you have a corn allergy) are best.

EGGS

Choose free-range. They are available in most supermarkets. Eggs have had a bad press lately but properly cooked they are a useful part of the candida diet. They are full of essential nutrients and research has shown (*Mental and Elemental Nutrients* Carl C. Pfeiffer, published by Keats Publishing, Inc, 1975) that the high sulphur content in eggs helps to control fungus in the gut. Dr Pfeiffer encourages people without a history of heart disease or high blood pressure to use eggs freely in the diet. As far as cholesterol goes there are many foods which people happily include in their diet, such as pastries, cakes, sausage rolls and hamburgers which are just as high in fat and which do not provide the essential nutrients found in the egg.

CEREALS

Throw out all commercial cereals including muesli which contain sugar and any flour or cereal which has been lurking in the cupboard for some time.

WHEAT

If you have a severe candida problem and particularly if you are overweight you would be better to avoid wheat products altogether for at least three months. My experience is that severe candida sufferers invariably have a wheat intolerance and they are much better without it. It can be introduced once in four days when the symptoms abate. Foods you have eaten regularly all your life are the ones which are most likely to cause you problems. For more information read *Coping with Candida* (see Further Reading, page 139).

If you lose weight when you give up bread, despite eating more rice, potatoes and other complex carbohydrates, it would be advisable to seek professional help.

Alternatives to Wheat

So many people panic and think they will starve if they

give up bread. There are plenty of alternative grains. They include: rice, oats, rye, buckwheat, millet, barley, quinoa (this is an ancient grain prized by the Incas – it looks like small sago but has a better flavour), sago, tapioca.

Couscous is a wheat product but some people who react to other wheat products seem to tolerate this. It comes precooked and only needs to be soaked in boiling water and covered for seven minutes before serving. It is a delicious alternative to rice.

Alternatives to Wheat Flour

Most of the above grains can be found as flour and in addition there is potato flour, soybean flour, gram flour (made from chick peas), cornflour, maize meal. Arrowroot can be used in baking and for thickening soups, stews and sauces. A grated or mashed potato, or a table-spoonful of instant potato can also be used for thickening. Use these in the recipes in preference to wheat.

PULSES

Dried beans, peas, chick peas, and lentils are cheap and nutritious and for many people provide many of the main meals of their anticandida diet. There are however a few points to consider. Since they contain both protein and starch, people who are more comfortable when they eat starches and proteins at different times find them indigestible. For further information, read *Food Combining for Health – Don't Mix Foods That Fight* (see Further Reading, page 138). Long soaking makes them more digestible, particularly if you leave whole seeds long enough to sprout. This also increases their food value. Red lentils cook quite quickly and do not really need soaking from this point of view, but soaking overnight does help to stop them producing so much gas in the intestine.

Soaking Pulses

These can be left on the kitchen windowsill in bowls of cold water for several days. Change the water twice each day. It is exciting to see the shoots appearing from withered looking seeds and realize that they are living, fresh foods. Mung beans will sprout in a few days but the larger seeds like chick peas take longer. If you are not ready to use the sprouted beans or seeds, drain them and keep them in a plastic bag in the refrigerator. They will keep fresh (and amazingly keep growing) for several days. Do not eat raw sprouted red kidney or aduki beans. They contain substances which are destroyed by cooking but are poisonous when eaten raw.

Long soaking greatly reduces cooking time, makes them more nutritious and digestible. Adding a piece of kombu (seaweed) (see Sea Vegetables page 21) to pulses flavours, adds nutrients and tenderizes them.

For full instructions on sprouting seeds and pulses, their value to health, and delicious recipes read *Raw Energy* (see Further Reading, page 138).

DAIRY PRODUCTS

Some practitioners exclude all dairy products. Others allow live yogurt and cottage cheese. Persons with intolerance to cows' milk can often tolerate moderate amounts of evaporated milk. The fat in milk is less likely to cause trouble than the milk sugar and milk protein, and in fact some people feel they can tolerate whole milk better than skimmed milk. Some cows' milk intolerant people have no trouble with goats' milk or goats' milk products. The milk is available frozen and dried in health food stores. Milk is a mucous-forming food and if you have catarrhal symptoms you would be better without it. Soya milk is widely used as a milk alternative and is available in some supermarkets as well as health food stores. Non-milk vegetable 'creamers' can also be used.

DRINKS

All drinks containing sugar are out, even if your symptoms are improving. If this makes you cut down on tea and coffee so much the better. Moderate use of artificial sweeteners is allowed but it's better if you can avoid overuse of these as they perpetuate the taste for sweet drinks and contain additives.

Alcohol

Alcohol feeds candida and disturbs the blood sugar levels. Avoid completely if your symptoms are severe and in the first few weeks of treatment.

Fruit juices

Only freshly squeezed juices – the cartons contain yeasts. Soft drinks all contain citric acid which is a form of yeast. So many 'cystitis' sufferers lose their symptoms when they stop drinking cartons of fruit juice and soft drinks.

Treats when your symptoms are under control: A daily glass of dry white wine, a diet drink, 1 gin or vodka with a diet mixer. A hot chocolate diet drink.

Drinks made from spring water, fruit juices and herbs without added sugar can be taken more freely.

Tea and Coffee

Some people feel a great deal better when they stop these altogether (if you do this watch out for the 'caffeine storm' – see Further Reading (page 138), *Coping with Candida*). Others find this difficult and just try to cut down. Herb teas can be soothing and refreshing. Pau Darco, a strong antifungal tea is available from New Nutrition (see Useful Addresses, page 142).

OIL

Olive oil is best not only because it prevents the yeast cell progressing to its invasive form but also because it helps to lower cholesterol levels and is safer when heated than other oils (although it should not be heated to smoking point). Cold-pressed virgin oil is best because its processing does not involve heating. Its drawback is that some people find the taste too strong. The lighter olive oil is almost tasteless but being more processed may not give the same benefits as the cold-pressed oil. Cold-pressed oils contain essential fatty acids which the body can easily absorb. Sunflower, sesame and walnut oils are good choices particularly for salads. Corn and safflower oils can also be used, but avoid mixed vegetable oils which might be cheaper but will be less pure and may have lost more in the processing.

ANIMAL FATS

After years of being told by scientists to eat margarine we are now being told butter is safer because the heating necessary in the production of margarine produces chemicals the body can't cope with. Butter tastes very much better anyway. You will notice I have used it in the recipes. Fat has always been a natural part of man's diet. It is sugar and refined carbohydrates that are unnatural. Perhaps it is the combination of these rather than the fat alone which cause so many of the illnesses of modern man. It is not necessary to worry too much about fat on the candida diet, in fact better if you include a little more if you have always been careful about this. Research in America showed an increased risk of acute depression and suicide in women on very low fat diets. Besides, you will be eating lots of foods (vegetables, garlic, onions, apples) that actually lower the cholesterol levels. A report in the Observer Magazine some years ago entitled 'The Stinker with A Heart Of Gold', stated that if a raw onion was eaten after eating a bacon and egg breakfast the cholesterol levels were actually lower than before the breakfast had been consumed.

SALT

Whilst it is not healthy to sprinkle liberal amounts of salt on your food (particularly if you have high blood pressure, heart problems or suffer from fluid retention), unless your doctor has put you on a low salt diet a little sea salt (better than table salt because it contains trace elements) in cooking is acceptable – and even advisable if you have low blood pressure (a condition that goes unnoticed here but not in France where moderate amounts of salt and coffee are recommended).

SEA VEGETABLES (SEAWEED)

These are available in dried form in health food stores. They are a very useful addition to the anticandida diet. The carbohydrate from them is not absorbed and they are rich in mineral and trace elements. Scientific research (Dr Tanaka of McGill University in Canada) has proven that the glutinous part of seaweed bonds with heavy metal pollutants such as mercury and lead in the intestines and prevents them being absorbed. Sea vegetables come dried in flat packets with full instructions on how to use them. Don't be put off by the strange names; try them in soups, stews and salads or toasted and sprinkled on vegetables. They include nori, arame, kombu, wakame, sea palm and dulse. Agar flakes can be used as gelatine. Since quite small quantities are used, and they keep well, they are an inexpensive addition to your store-cupboard.

ADDITIVES

Read about these. There will be books in your local library. Many are to be avoided but they are not all harmful. You could make a list of the undesirable ones and keep it in your purse. It should not be too much of a worry since you will not be eating many prepared foods.

Recipe Notes

- Recipes serve 2 unless otherwise stated
- Follow either metric or imperial measures for the recipes in this book as they are not interchangeable
- All spoon measures are level unless otherwise stated
- Size 2 free-range eggs should be used unless otherwise stated
- Milk is semi-skimmed unless otherwise stated
- Plain flour is used unless otherwise stated

COOKING TERMS

Aubergine	Eggplant
Baking tray	Cookie sheet
Beetroot	Beets
Bicarbonate of soda	Baking soda
Biscuits, savoury	Crackers
Biscuits, sweet	Cookies
Black olives	Ripe olives
Broad beans	Fava beans, or use lima beans
Butter muslin	Cheesecloth
Cake mixture	Cake batter
Cake tin	Cake pan
Chillies, green/red	Chili peppers
Chick peas	Garbanzos
Chicory	Belgian endive
Cocktail stick	Toothpick
Coriander	Cilantro
Cornflour	Cornstarch
Cos lettuce	Romaine
Cottage cheese	Pot cheese
Courgettes	Zucchini
Curly endive	Chicory
Dessert apples	Eating apples
Digestive biscuits	Use graham crackers
Double cream	Heavy/whipping cream
Essence	Extract
Flaked almonds	Slivered almonds
Frying pan	Skillet
Grated rind	Grated zest or peel

Candida Albicans

Greaseproof paper	Waxed paper
Grill/grilled	Broil/broiled
Groundnut oil	Peanut oil
Gruyere cheese	Swiss cheese
Haricot beans	Navy beans
Heart of lettuce	Bulk of Boston lettuce
Maize flour	Corn meal
Mange tout	Snow peas
Marrow	Large zucchini/marrow squash
Minced beef	Ground beef
Mixture	Batter
Pearl barley	Pot barley
Pepper, green/red	Sweet bell pepper
Plaice	Flounder
Porridge oats	Rolled/quick cookingoats
Scones	Biscuits
Single cream	Light cream
Soya beans	Soybeans
Spring onion	Scallion
Stoned	Pitted
Sultanas	Golden raisins
Swede	Rutabaga
Tomato purée	Tomato paste
Walnuts	English walnuts
Wholewheat plain flour	Whole-wheat flour
Wholewheat self-raising flour	Whole-wheat flour sifted with baking powder
Yeast, dried	Active-dry yeast
Yeast, fresh	Compressed yeast

2

Good Stock Is Essential

THE DAYS are long-gone when there was always a
pot of stock simmering away on the stove. If you
have time and enjoy cooking, why not recall those days
and make your own stocks? There is not a lot of effort
involved, and they can be made at any time and frozen for
when you need them.

Be adventurous with your stocks: throw in your leftovers such as scrubbed vegetable peelings and any
undressed salad you have, and try experimenting with
more herbs and spices.

If you need to buy stock rather than make your own,
excellent vegetable and meat stock cubes are available in
most supermarkets. More unusual ones such as French
onion and tomato can be found in health food stores where
you will also find vegetable stock powder. This is free of
yeast, colouring and additives and there is also a low salt
variety. It is convenient to use and more versatile than cubes
since it can be sprinkled on salads and steamed vegetables.

Use the following recipes as guidelines for home-
made stock.

VEGETABLE STOCK (1)

Metric/Imperial		*American*
900g/2lb	mixed vegetables	2lb
	(eg cabbage, root vegetables,	
	leeks, onions, shallots, garlic,	
	celery (plus tops), peppers,	
	courgettes (zucchini),	
	tomatoes, celeriac, peas,	
	beans	

1. Put the vegetables, herbs and salt in a large saucepan. Cover with cold water and bring to the boil. Cover and simmer for 1 hour. Leave to cool then strain.
2. If you want a thicker stock rub some of the vegetables through a sieve.

VEGETABLE STOCK (2)

Roasting the vegetables before simmering brings out the natural sugars and gives a much fuller flavour to the stock. Peppers, for instance, taste entirely different when they are roasted. Onions, garlic and shallots can be roasted in their skins. Hard white cabbage can be quartered – trim the discoloured part of the stalk and leave the rest. Leave courgettes whole unless they are very large. Root vegetables do not need peeling. Scrub and roughly chop.

1. Put the vegetables on an oiled baking tray in a preheated oven at 200°C/400°F/gas mark 6 for about 1 hour. Baste at intervals and remove any that are in danger of becoming too brown. Transfer to a large pan and simmer as above.

MEAT STOCK

Metric/Imperial		American
900g/2 lb	meat bones (beef, lamb, pork or a mixture)	2 lb
2 large	onions (or 1 large leek), roughly chopped	2 large
6	garlic cloves, unpeeled and squashed	6
1 large	carrot, scrubbed and roughly chopped	1 large
¼	swede (or 2 white turnips), scrubbed and roughly chopped	¼
2 sticks	celery	2 stalks
	any other vegetables you have	
	water to cover	
5	black peppercorns	5
1½ tsp	salt	1½ tsp
1	bayleaf	1
	any fresh or dried herbs you wish (eg thyme, parsley)	

1. First roast the vegetables and bones in a preheated oven at 200°C/400°F/gas mark 6 until they are browned and the juices are running, then place in a large saucepan and cover with water. Add the remaining ingredients and simmer for 2½–3 hours.
2. Strain, cool then refrigerate. The fat will form a hard layer on top, which should be removed.

Good Stock Is Essential

CHICKEN STOCK (1)

Metric/Imperial		American
1	chicken carcass	1
1 large	carrot, roughly chopped	1 large
1 large	onion, roughly chopped	1 large
2 sticks	celery (or ½ tsp celery seed)	2 stalks
1 tsp	dried sage (or large sprig of fresh sage)	1 tsp
1 tsp	salt	1 tsp

1. Put all the ingredients in a large saucepan, cover with cold water and bring to the boil. Cover and simmer for about 1½ hours.
2. Strain, add any meat left on the carcass, then cool and refrigerate. Remove the fat that forms on the top.

CHICKEN STOCK (2)

Metric/Imperial		American
1	whole boiling chicken, about 900g–1kg/ 2–2½ lb	1
1 large	onion	1 large
6	garlic cloves	6
1½ tsp	salt	1½ tsp
½ tsp	freshly ground black pepper	½ tsp
2.8 litres/ 5 pints	water	13 cups

1. Wash the chicken and remove excess fat.
2. Put all the ingredients in a large saucepan and bring to the boil. Cover and simmer for 3¼–4 hours (check there is always enough water to cover the bird). Strain and allow to cool.
3. Much of the chicken disintegrates and produces a jelly-like rich stock. When cool rub as much of this as you can through a sieve. Stir in a little cold water so that the fat can rise to the surface, then refrigerate. Remove the fat that forms on top.
4. Divide the stock into four portions to freeze. Each portion will be enough stock for soup for two. You might need to add a little water to the soup when adding your vegetables, noodles, rice etc.

FISH STOCK

Fish stock cubes are available but so far I have not found one with the flavour of a home-made stock. They also tend to be very salty. The Chinese make wonderful fish stock, so it could be worth looking in a Chinese super-market. Check for additives and yeast.

Metric/Imperial		American
900g/2 lb	white fish head, shoulders or bones	2 lb
1.1 litres/ 2 pints	water	5 cups
1	lemon, juice of	1
1 tsp	salt	1 tsp
bunch	spring onions (or 6 shallots)	bunch
½ tsp	dried (or handful of chopped fresh) dill or fennel	½ tsp
handful	chopped fresh parsley	handful

1. Wash the fish and bones carefully. Any blood left will give the stock a bitter taste.
2. Put all the ingredients in a large saucepan, cover and simmer gently for 30 minutes. Do not overcook as this will also make it bitter. Strain, cool and store.

3

Good Soup Is Easy

SOUP IS A USEFUL part of the candida diet. It is nutritious and low in carbohydrate. Thick soups can be taken as main meals and thin soups taken before a meal can give a feeling of fullness which prevents cravings for dessert. Thick soups can be frozen in freezer bags and thin ones in well-washed large yogurt cartons – keep them upright until they are frozen solid.

RED LENTIL SOUP

Metric/Imperial		American
100g/4oz	red lentils, washed	½ cup
2	carrots, scrubbed and grated	2
1	potato, scrubbed and grated	1
1 small	leek, finely chopped	1 small
2 tsp	vegetable stock powder (or 1 vegetable stock cube or ½ tsp salt)	2 tsp
	chopped fresh parsley or coriander, to garnish	

1. Put all the ingredients in a saucepan and cover with water to about 5cm/2 inches above the vegetables.
2. Bring to the boil, cover and simmer until cooked. This will take 45 minutes if the lentils have been soaked, or 1–1¼ hours if not. Stir occasionally to prevent 'catching' and add more water if it is becoming too thick.
3. Garnish with chopped fresh parsley or coriander.

PARSNIP SOUP

Metric/Imperial		American
1	onion	1
1	potato, diced	1
1 tbsp	olive oil	1 tbsp
600ml/1 pint	vegetable or chicken stock	2½ cups
680g/1½ lb	parsnips, peeled and diced	1½ lb
½	lemon, juice of	½
½ tsp	dried sage (or 6 fresh sage leaves)	½ tsp
	a little milk (optional)	
	yogurt or single cream and toasted sesame seeds, to serve	

1. Gently sauté the onion and potato in the oil for about 10 minutes, but do not brown.
2. Add the stock and remaining ingredients, cover and simmer for 30 minutes. Blend or rub through a sieve and reheat.
3. Add a little milk, or milk substitute if you feel it is too thick.
4. Serve with a spoonful of yogurt or single cream in the middle of the bowl, and sprinkle with toasted sesame seeds.

Variation

Omit the sage and add 1 heaped tsp curry powder when sautéing onions and potatoes. Serve with toasted cumin seeds.

SCOTCH BROTH

This is a less complicated version of the traditional recipe. It is a hearty soup suitable for a main course.

If you want to lower the fat content add a little cold water at the end of the cooking time to make it easier to skim, then reheat. If you are not using the soup immediately, cool and refrigerate overnight. Make sure the ingredients are submerged in the liquid, then the fat can easily be lifted off with a spoon.

Metric/Imperial		American
225g/8oz	stewing lamb	½ lb
1.1 litres/ 2 pints	water	5 cups
1½	stock cubes (lamb, chicken or vegetable or 3½ tsp vegetable stock powder)	1½
1 medium	onion, diced	1 medium
50g/2oz	pearl barley (soaked overnight)	¼ cup
1 large	potato, scrubbed and diced	1 large
2	carrots, scrubbed and diced	2
50g/2oz	dried peas (soaked overnight)	¼ cup

1. Trim the fat from lamb, and cut into 1 cm/½ inch cubes.
2. Put all the ingredients in a large saucepan, and bring to the boil. Cover and simmer for 1½–2 hours or until the peas are cooked.

JUICED TOMATO SOUP
WITH GARLIC CROUTONS

This can be made in 5 minutes if you have a juicer.

Metric/Imperial		American
6	tomatoes	6
2	carrots, scrubbed	2
2 tbsp	cooked peas	2 tbsp
handful	chopped fresh chives or spring onions	handful
	boiling water	
	pinch of salt	

Croutons		
1 slice	wholemeal or wheatfree bread, cubed	1 slice
3	garlic cloves, crushed	3
	olive oil, for frying	

1. Juice the carrots and tomatoes and pour into a saucepan.
2. Add the remaining ingredients and simmer for 5 minutes.
3. To make the croutons, sauté the garlic in olive oil for 5 minutes. The oil will then be flavoured.
4. Remove the garlic, raise the heat and fry the bread cubes until golden brown. Drain on kitchen paper, then serve with the soup.

CREAMED CAULIFLOWER SOUP

Metric/Imperial		American
knob	butter or margarine (or 1 tbsp vegetable oil)	knob
1	onion, finely chopped	1
1 small	cauliflower, greens and stalk included, roughly chopped	1 small
600ml/1 pint	vegetable stock (or 1½ tsp stock powder)	2½ cups

1. Heat the butter or oil in a saucepan and sauté the onion until soft and light golden.
2. Add the cauliflower and stock and bring to the boil. Stir, then cover and simmer for 30 minutes.
3. Blend or rub through a sieve.
4. Taste and adjust the seasoning and reheat.

Serving Suggestions:

Spoonful of yogurt or single cream in the middle of each bowl; grated nutmeg; roasted sesame seeds; chopped fresh chives or spring onions; crunchy onion rings; sprinkling of roasted sea vegetables such as dulse or nori.

CORIANDER SOUP

Recipes which say if you can't find coriander, use parsley, baffle me. The flavour is completely different. Admittedly the appearance is similar – that of a broad-leafed parsley. Bunches of fresh coriander are available at many Asian stores – my advice on this one is wait until you have found one before you try this recipe. This is a quick soup with a unique flavour.

Metric/Imperial		American
50g/2oz	diced potato	⅓ cup
1 small	onion, diced	1 small
600ml/1 pint	vegetable or chicken stock	2½ cups
piece	fresh ginger root, grated (about half the size of your thumb)	piece
½ tsp	ground coriander	½ tsp
1 tsp	ground cumin	1 tsp
4 tbsp	chopped fresh coriander	4 tbsp
¼	fresh green chilli, finely chopped	¼
175g/6oz	frozen or fresh green peas	¾ cup
2 tsp	lemon juice	2 tsp

To serve:

1 tbsp	single cream or plain yogurt	1 tbsp
	roasted cumin seeds	
	finely chopped fresh coriander	

1. Put all the ingredients in a saucepan. Bring to the boil, cover and simmer for 20 minutes.
2. Blend or rub through a sieve (or you can press the vegetables with a potato masher).
3. Serve with the cream or yogurt in the middle of the soup, and sprinkle with roasted cumin seeds and chopped fresh coriander.

TOMATO SOUP

Metric/Imperial		American
1 tbsp	olive oil (or knob of butter or margarine)	1 tbsp
1	potato, scrubbed and diced	1
1	onion, finely chopped	1
450g/1 lb	tomatoes, finely chopped	1 lb
1	carrot, scrubbed and diced	1
1 tbsp	tomato purée	1 tbsp
600ml/1 pint	vegetable stock	2½ cups
sprig	fresh basil (or ½ tsp dried basil)	sprig
1 tsp	cornflour or arrowroot	1 tsp
a little	milk, or milk substitute	a little
	chopped fresh herbs (basil, parsley, coriander or chives) to serve	

1. Heat the oil or butter in a saucepan and sauté the potato and onion for 5 minutes.
2. Add the remaining ingredients, cover and simmer for 25 minutes.
3. Blend or rub through a sieve, then return to the pan to reheat.
4. To thicken, blend the cornflour or arrowroot with the milk or milk substitute. Add to the soup and cook gently, stirring all the time.
5. Serve with chopped fresh herbs scattered on top.

CHICKEN SOUP

Metric/Imperial		American
1 tbsp	olive oil	1 tbsp
1 small	leek, finely chopped	1 small
2	garlic cloves, crushed	2
100g/4oz	sliced mushrooms (omit if you are sensitive to mushrooms)	1½ cups
1	chicken breast or leg (to provide about 100g/4oz/½ cup cooked chicken, diced)	1
1	potato, scrubbed and diced	1
1	carrot, scrubbed and diced	1
50g/2oz	peas (frozen or fresh)	⅓ cup
50g/2oz	sweetcorn (frozen, fresh or canned)	⅓ cup
1 stick	celery, finely chopped	1 stalk
1	chicken stock cube	1
	water to cover	
	chopped fresh or dried sage or marjoram, to serve	

1. Heat the oil in a saucepan and add the leeks, garlic, mushrooms and uncooked chicken (if using).
2. Add the remaining ingredients, cover and simmer for 30 minutes.
3. If using cooked chicken, add 5 minutes before the end of cooking time.

Candida Albicans

4. Serve with a sprinkling of chopped fresh or dried sage or marjoram.

Variation:

For a thicker soup add a large mashed potato, 2 tsp arrowroot or cornflour blended with 2 tbsp milk or milk substitute. Simmer for 2 minutes.

DAVID'S CARROT AND LEMON SOUP

Metric/Imperial		American
2	carrots, grated	2
1	lemon, grated zest of (and juice of ½)	1
piece	fresh ginger root, grated (about the size of a large thumb)	piece
1 tsp	vegetable stock powder	1 tsp
600ml/1 pint	water	2½ cups
	chopped fresh chives, to serve	

1. Put all the ingredients in a saucepan. Bring to the boil, cover and simmer for 20 minutes.
2. Serve with a sprinkling of chopped fresh chives.

CREAMY FISH SOUP

Metric/Imperial		American
900g/2 lb	cod shoulder (or 450g/1 lb cod cheeks, or any white fish)	2 lb
1	onion, roughly chopped	1
1	carrot, scrubbed and roughly chopped	1
¼ tsp	salt	¼ tsp
4	black peppercorns (or black pepper to taste)	4
1	potato, diced	1
2 tbsp	peas (fresh or frozen)	2 tbsp
2 tbsp	sweetcorn (fresh, frozen or canned)	2 tbsp
handful	fresh parsley, finely chopped	handful
2 tbsp	powdered milk (or 4 tbsp single cream)	2 tbsp
2 tsp	arrowroot or cornflour (omit if using cream)	2 tsp

1. Wash the fish. Put in a saucepan with the onion, carrot and seasoning, and cover with cold water.
2. Simmer for 20 minutes, then strain, reserving stock (you should have about 1 pint/600ml).
3. Return the stock to the pan. Flake the flesh off the fish and add to the pan with the potatoes, peas and sweetcorn. Simmer until the potatoes are tender.

4. Add the parsley to the pan. Blend the milk and arrow-root with a little cold water and stir into the soup until thickened. Alternatively, add the cream.
5. If your diet is milk-free, blend arrowroot with soya milk or thicken the soup with mashed or instant potato.

ROCK POOL SOUP

This is a clear, delicately flavoured dark green soup. My family gave it the above name.

Metric/Imperial		American
25g/1oz	sea vegetable (eg nori, wakame, arame)	2 tbsp
3 handfuls	fine strips of spring greens	3 handfuls
small bunch	spring onions, halved horizontally, finely sliced lengthways	small bunch
1	French onion stock cube	1
¼	unpeeled cucumber, cut into thin strips	¼
25g/1oz	rice noodles	2 tbsp
750ml/1¼ pints	water	3 cups
100g/4oz	cooked shrimps, crab meat monkfish, or any cooked white fish	⅔ cup
	chopped spring onions to garnish	

1. Soak the sea vegetables for 10 minutes. Roll up like a cigar and cut with scissors into fine strips.
2. Place all the ingredients, except the fish, in boiling water and simmer for 15 minutes.
3. Add the fish 2 minutes before serving.
4. Garnish with chopped spring onions.

4

Why Raw Vegetables?

THE VALUE OF fresh raw vegetables to health cannot be overemphasized. Many people think if they eat salad sandwiches or have a lettuce and tomato salad with cold meat, or tuna a couple of times a week, that they have an adequate intake of raw food. The idea of eating a main course consisting entirely of raw vegetables is not considered a 'proper meal'.

People with digestive problems often say 'But I couldn't possibly eat raw vegetables, I have enough trouble eating them cooked.' The same people are often astonished at the improvement in their digestion when they gradually introduce raw foods into their meals, and build up to a high raw diet. They start by eating a small quantity of raw vegetables, fruit or fruit juice before eating a cooked meal. There is a scientifically proven reason why this aids digestion.

Research done about sixty years ago at the Institute of Clinical Chemistry in Lausanne discovered that the body reacts to foods that have been altered by cooking and processing, and as a defence mechanism white blood cells pour into the intestines as soon as the food is chewed. This is called 'digestive leucocytosis'. White cells are a vital part of the body's defence against disease. If they are busy in the intestines several times a day it puts a strain on the immune system, and can be the start of lowered resistance to infection, allergies, and degenerative conditions such as arthritis. The reason why the white cell reaction is not triggered when you eat raw food could be that enzymes and acids necessary for the full absorption of the food have not been affected by heating and react normally with the saliva in the mouth. Chewing is a vital part of digestion: starches start to be broken down as they mix with the saliva. If food is bolted the first stage of digestion is lost, and not only does this prevent full absorption of the nutrients but also the result can be gas, a bloated abdomen and discomfort.

The research found that if something raw was eaten before a cooked meal digestive leucocytosis did not occur. It could be that the correct mechanism for good digestion is started by the raw food and then the body is better equipped to deal with the cooked food.

Even if you feel you could not cope with a high raw food diet, you could make a habit of eating some of the vegetables you are preparing for cooking or have some vegetable sticks with dips or a small salad before your meal. A small glass of freshly squeezed fruit juice (cans and cartons of juice should be avoided because they often contain yeasts) or a piece of apple or pear is also helpful.

DENTURES

People with dentures often say they find it difficult chewing raw foods. Grating food very finely and taking time over chewing overcomes this.

DIARRHOEA

People with frequent loose stools are concerned about raw foods making their diarrhoea worse. My experience is that well chewed raw foods rarely do this and in fact a great many sufferers find a high raw food diet helps. Permanent diarrhoea is unpleasant and debilitating. If your doctor can find no organic reason for the condition then you are clearly eating something that is irritating your bowel or else you are nervously exhausted through worrying too much. Diarrhoea is an attempt by the bowel to flush out a substance it finds unacceptable. It could be that you have developed some food intolerances. (For further reading, see *The Irritable Bowel and Diverticulosis* published by Thorsons, or *Coping With Candida* published by Sheldon Press, both by the writer.)

MORE REASONS FOR A HIGH RAW FOOD DIET

1. Primitive cultures eating fresh raw foods untainted by pesticides have been found to be virtually free from dental caries and many of the degenerative diseases, such as arthritis and cancer,

which are endemic in the modern world.

2. Raw foods detoxify the body not only by the action of certain enzymes but also by providing fibre. This keeps the muscles in the bowel wall healthy which in turn increases peristalis (the movement which pushes the faeces through the bowel), therefore the transit time is less and this prevents putrefaction and the breeding of harmful bacteria and fungi. Vegetable fibre is less irritating to the bowel than cereal fibre. Bran with everything is not a good idea: bran is for horses!

3. Raw foods promote healing by enhancing the action of the enzymes produced in the body.

4. A clean bowel is able to produce the B vitamins and vitamin K.

5. The cellulose in raw vegetables swells and gives a feeling of fullness which is useful for weight control. It also helps control blood sugar levels. See *Coping Successfully with Panic Attacks* by the author and published by Sheldon, for more on why it is important to keep blood sugar levels stable.

THE RECIPES

The recipes in this chapter demonstrate the versatility of raw ingredients, while taking the time to make tasty dips for vegetable sticks and dressings for salads will make a high raw food diet more interesting.

MAYONNAISE

Makes about 240ml/8floz

Metric/Imperial		American
2	egg yolks	2
2 tbsp	lemon juice	2 tbsp
1 tsp	mustard powder	1 tsp
½ tsp	vegetable stock powder	½ tsp
	(or ¼ tsp salt)	
	freshly ground black pepper,	
	to taste	
160ml/6fl oz	olive oil, light olive oil or	¾ cup
	sunflower oil	

1. Combine all the ingredients except the oil.
2. Slowly drizzle in the oil, beating with a wooden spoon (or if using a blender, slowly add the oil through the hole in the lid).
3. Store in the fridge in a screwtop jar. Will keep for 4 days.

Variations:

Garlic mayonnaise – add 2–4 cloves crushed garlic.

Tarragon mayonnaise – add 2 tbsp finely chopped fresh tarragon (French has the best aniseed flavour) or 1 tbsp dried tarragon.

Herb mayonnaise – add a large handful of any fresh herbs you have finely chopped.

Hot mayonnaise – ¼ finely chopped red or green pepper or ¼ tsp chilli powder.

Avocado mayonnaise – blend in 1 ripe avocado.

Candida Albicans

TAHINI MAYONNAISE

Metric/Imperial		American
2	garlic cloves, crushed	2
½ tsp	vegetable stock powder (or ¼ tsp salt)	½ tsp
3 tbsp	tahini (ground sesame seeds available in jars from healthfood stores)	3 tbsp
2 tbsp	cold water	2 tbsp
1	lemon, juice of	1

1. Stir the garlic and vegetable stock powder or salt into the tahini.
2. Blend in the water and lemon juice a little at a time, using a blender or in a mixing bowl.
3. Store in the fridge in a screwtop jar.

FRENCH DRESSING

Metric/Imperial		American
6 tbsp	oil	6 tbsp
2 tbsp	lemon juice	2 tbsp
½ tsp	mustard powder	½ tsp
1 tsp	honey (optional)	1 tsp
½ tsp	vegetable stock powder	½ tsp
	(or ¼ tsp salt)	

1. Put all the ingredients into a clean screwtop jar and shake until emulsified. Will keep for about 1 week in the fridge.

Variations:

Garlic dressing – add 3 crushed cloves of garlic.

Herb dressing – add a handful of finely chopped fresh herbs.

Dried mint dressing – add 1 heaped tbsp dried mint.

YOGURT DIP

Makes 125ml/4floz

Metric/Imperial		American
Metric/Imperial		*American*
6 tbsp	plain yogurt	6 tbsp
2	garlic cloves, crushed	2
2 tsp	olive oil	2 tsp
large pinch	salt	large pinch
	freshly ground black pepper, to taste	

1. Combine all the ingredients by hand or in a blender.

Variations:

Curry dip – omit the garlic and add ½ tsp curry powder and 1 dsp desiccated coconut.

Mint and cucumber dip – add quarter of a grated cucumber and 1 dsp of dried mint or a handful of finely chopped fresh mint.

Seed dip – add 2 tsp dry-roasted cumin or caraway seeds.

Mustard dip – add ½ tsp dried mustard powder.

Onion and paprika dip – add ½ grated onion, 1 dsp paprika, dash of Tabasco sauce (optional).

Herb dip – add a handful of finely chopped fresh herbs; chives, thyme, sage, basil, mint or anything you have.

HUMOUS

Metric/Imperial		American
100g/4oz	chick peas, soaked overnight and drained	½ cup
900ml/1½ pints	water	3¾ cups
1 tsp	salt	1 tsp
1 tbsp	tahini (ground sesame seeds available in jars from healthfood stores)	1 tbsp
1	lemon, juice of	1
3	garlic cloves, crushed	3

1. Simmer the chick peas in the water for 1 hour. Add the salt and simmer until tender.
2. Drain, and reserve the cooking water.
3. Blend the cooked chick peas with 125ml/4floz reserved cooking water in a blender, or rub the chick peas through a sieve and add the water.
4. Mix in the remaining ingredients and refrigerate.
5. Use either as a dip for raw vegetables or smooth into individual portions in shallow bowls. Make a well in the centre and pour in a little olive oil. Sprinkle with paprika and chopped parsley.
6. Serve with warm yeast-free pitta bread.

Note:

To freeze – well-washed yogurt cartons with lids are convenient storage containers.

COLESLAW

If you are in a hurry use commercial mayonnaise and plain yogurt in equal quantities.

Metric/Imperial		American
1	garlic clove, lightly crushed plus as much chopped garlic as you like (optional)	1
½	white cabbage, finely shredded	½
1	carrot, grated	1
1 stick	celery, chopped	1 stalk
2	dessert apples, peeled, cored and chopped	2
1 small	onion (or 2 shallots), finely chopped	1 small
50g/2oz	pumpkin or sesame seeds (optional)	¼ cup
125ml/4fl oz	Yogurt Dips (page 55)	½ cup
125ml/4fl oz	Mayonnaise (page 52)	½ cup

1. Rub the lightly crushed garlic clove around a large salad bowl.
2. Place the vegetables and seeds in the bowl. Mix together the dressings and stir into the vegetables.

NUTTY RED CABBAGE

Metric/Imperial		American
100g/4oz	cashew nuts	¾ cup
	oil or butter, for frying	
½	red cabbage, grated	½
2	dessert apples, peeled and grated	2
½	lemon, juice and grated zest	½
4 tbsp	plain yogurt	4 tbsp
pinch	salt	pinch

1. Fry the cashew nuts in a little oil or butter until golden brown, then lift out with a slotted spoon.
2. Combine the remaining ingredients in a bowl and stir in the nuts.

PEPPERY SALAD

Metric/Imperial		American
1	carrot, grated	1
1cm/½ inch slice	swede, grated	½ inch slice
1 small	parsnip, grated	1 small
6	radishes, chopped or 2 tbsp grated mouli (white radish)	6
	Mayonnaise (page 52)	
	watercress, to garnish	

1. Combine all the vegetables, and stir in enough mayonnaise to coat.
2. Serve garnished with sprigs of watercress.

AVOCADO AND WATERCRESS SALAD

The avocado should feel like a ripe pear. If it does not yield to the touch leave it in a warm place for a couple of days. They are pretty tasteless unless they are ripe.

Metric/Imperial		American
1	ripe avocado	1
¼	iceberg lettuce, torn into small pieces	¼
bunch	watercress, separated into small pieces	bunch
	French Dressing (page 54)	
	pumpkin seeds, to garnish	

1. Halve the avocado lengthways around the stone and separate. Remove the stone by tapping it with the middle of the blade of a sharp knife. The stone should stick to the knife and lift out easily.
2. Hold each half avocado in your palm and make several lengthways cuts and then cut across into dice. With a squeeze of the skin the pieces should fall out.
3. Mix the avocado with the lettuce and watercress, and toss in French dressing.
4. Garnish with pumpkin seeds to add a different texture.

PEPPER AND TOMATO SALAD

Metric/Imperial		American
½	green pepper, cored and seeded	½
½	red pepper, cored and seeded	½
2 large	tomatoes	2 large
6	black olives	6
	French Dressing (page 54) or Herb Dressing (page 54)	
sprinkling	vegetable stock powder (optional)	sprinkling

1. Slice the peppers into thin rings, then quarter the slices.
2. Slice the tomatoes, then quarter the slices.
3. Halve and stone the olives.
4. Toss the salad in the dressing with the vegetable stock powder (if using).

CARROT AND BEETROOT SALAD

Most people do not think of eating raw beetroot. Try it with carrots. It is very cleansing and has a tangy flavour.

Metric/Imperial		*American*
1 small	fresh, raw beetroot	1 small
2	carrots	2
	French Dressing (page 54)	
	to serve	

1. Peel and grate the beetroot.
2. Scrub and grate the carrots.
3. Combine the vegetables and serve with the dressing.

CARROT SALAD

Metric/Imperial		American
1 tsp	black mustard seeds	1 tsp
2 tbsp	olive oil	2 tbsp
2	garlic cloves, crushed	2
2	carrots, scrubbed and grated	2

1. Fry the mustard seeds in hot oil for about 1 minute.
2. Add the garlic and fry until golden brown.
3. Pour the oil mixture over the grated carrots, and serve immediately.

BEETROOT SALAD

Many people reach for prepacked cooked beetroot instead of cooking it themselves. There is not much effort involved and it tastes much better this way.

Metric/Imperial		American
2	beetroot (about 250g/½ lb)	2
	water to cover	
2 tbsp	olive oil	2 tbsp
¼ tsp	salt	¼ tsp
large handful	finely chopped fresh parsley or coriander	large handful

1. Trim the leaves from the beetroot, but do not peel or top and tail.
2. Boil for 30–45 minutes. Test with sharp pointed knife. This should slip in and out easily when the beetroot is tender.
3. Remove the skin under cold running water, and top and tail.
4. Slice and dice the beetroot, then mix with the oil and sprinkle with the salt and parsley.
5. Serve hot or cold.

Variation:

Serve beetroot hot with a knob of butter. It goes well with fish and broad beans or lentil dishes.

TOMATOES WITH FRESH BASIL

Metric/Imperial		American
4	tomatoes	4
½ small	onion (or 2 shallots)	½ small
12	basil leaves	12
	salt, pepper and sugar	
1 tbsp	olive oil	1 tbsp
squeeze	lemon juice	squeeze

1. Chop the tomatoes. Peel and finely chop the onion or shallots. Shred the basil leaves.
2. Combine the ingredients in a bowl, season with a little salt and pepper and a pinch of sugar. Add the oil and lemon juice and lightly toss together.

Variation:

If you can't find fresh basil, use 2 tbsp chopped fresh coriander, mint or chives.

CELERY AND APPLE SALAD

Metric/Imperial		American
1	head celery	1
2	dessert apples	2
50g/2oz	walnuts, chopped	½ cup
4 tbsp	Yogurt Dip (page 55) or Mayonnaise (page 52)	4 tbsp

1. Top and tail the celery (keep leaves for soup or coleslaw).
2. Wash the sticks of celery and bend in the middle until you reach the 'strings'. Pull the halves apart and most of the tough fibres can easily be pulled off. Chop into 2.5cm/1 inch pieces.
3. Peel, core and dice the apples.
4. Mix all the ingredients together.

Variations:

Cashew nuts, hazel nuts, pecan nuts, toasted pumpkin seeds or sunflower seeds can be used instead of walnuts.

SPINACH SALAD

Metric/Imperial		American
225g/8oz	fresh spinach	½ lb
2	hard-boiled egg yolks, finely chopped	2
2 rashers	bacon (optional), diced	2 slices
½	mild chilli, finely chopped (or ¼ tsp chilli powder)	½
2 tbsp	olive oil	2 tbsp

1. Wash the spinach as soon as possible after purchase, and soak for 30 minutes in cold water. This should make it really crisp. Shake it dry and put in a plastic bag in the fridge. It should keep quite well for a day or two if you don't need it immediately.
2. Fry the bacon and chilli in the hot oil.
3. Break the spinach into bite-size pieces and put in a serving bowl.
4. Remove the pan from the heat and quickly blend in the egg yolks.
5. Pour the mixture over the spinach and serve immediately.

HOT POTATO SALAD

Metric/Imperial		American
3	potatoes	3
	salt	
4 tbsp	plain yogurt	4 tbsp
1 tsp	cumin seeds	1 tsp
2	garlic cloves, finely chopped	2

1. Scrub the potatoes and chop into bite-size pieces.
2. Boil in salted water until tender.
3. Combine the yogurt, cumin and garlic in a bowl and mix in the potatoes. Serve hot.

MINTED POTATO SALAD

Metric/Imperial		American
3	potatoes	3
	salt	
2 tsp	dried mint	2 tsp
3 tbsp	plain yogurt	3 tbsp
2 tsp	olive oil	2 tsp

1. Scrub the potatoes and cook in salted water until tender. Cool and dice.
2. Blend the mint, yogurt and oil and season.
3. Mix with the potatoes, then refrigerate until needed.

FRENCH BEAN AND POTATO SALAD

Metric/Imperial		*American*
2	potatoes	2
225g/8oz	frozen or fresh French beans, chopped	2 cups
3 tbsp	Mayonnaise (page 52)	3 tbsp
10	anchovies, drained and chopped (optional)	10
1	hard-boiled egg (chopped)	1
1 tsp	capers, rinsed and chopped (optional)	1 tsp

1. Scrub the potatoes and chop into bite-size pieces.
2. Boil in salted water with the beans until tender. Drain and cool.
3. Mix the beans and potatoes with the mayonnaise and anchovies.
4. Top with the chopped hard-boiled egg and capers.

MIXED SPROUT SALAD

Metric/Imperial		American
175g/6oz	sprouted mung beans	3 cups
50g/2oz	sprouted sunflower seeds	1 cup
50g/2oz	sprouted pumpkin seeds	1 cup
	lettuce	
	Yogurt Dip (page 55) or	
	Mayonnaise (page 52)	

1. Combine all the sprouts and the dressing.
2. Serve on a bed of lettuce.

TUNA AND AVOCADO SALAD

Metric/Imperial		American
1	ripe avocado	1
2 sticks	celery	2 stalks
200g/7oz	canned tuna, drained	1 cup
	Mayonnaise (page 52),	
	for mixing	
	spinach leaves	
1	hard-boiled egg, chopped	1
	to garnish	

1. Peel and dice the avocado, and finely chop the celery.
2. Mix the tuna, celery and avocado with the mayonnaise, and serve on a bed of spinach.
3. Garnish with the chopped hard-boiled egg.

5

Vegetables Need Not Be Boring

COOKED AND RAW vegetables are going to be a large part of your anticandida diet. Get used to the idea that your shopping bag will be heavier. If you are without a car buy a haversack or shopping trolley.

This section concentrates on bringing out the natural sugars in vegetables. If you taste the cooking water of root vegetables or even greens you will be surprised by how sweet it is. You pour this natural sugar, vitamins and minerals down the kitchen sink when you boil vegetables. Steaming them preserves more nutrients and the flavour is somewhat improved but it cannot compare with the taste of vegetables prepared in ways that caramelize the natural sugars. There are several ways to do this: roasting in a little oil or water, stir-frying or water-'frying'. Most people only think of roasting potatoes but in fact all root vegetables, onions, leeks, courgettes, marrow, pumpkin, peppers, tomatoes and even hard cabbage can be cooked in this way and the extra time it takes is certainly worth it.

SIMPLE BAKED MIXED VEGETABLES

Metric/Imperial		American
2	carrots	2
2	parsnips	2
¼	swede	¼
1	red pepper	1
¼	hard white cabbage	¼
2 small (or 1 large)	courgettes	2 small (or 1 large)
1	leek (or 1 onion or 6 shallots or bulb of garlic)	1
	olive oil	
	stock	

1. Scrub and top and tail the carrots and parsnips and cut lengthways if large.
2. Cut the swede in two. The pepper can be roasted whole or halved, seeded and cooked cut side down.
3. Slice through the cabbage lengthways and also the courgettes if they are large. Small ones can be cooked whole.
4. Trim the leek, then cut lengthways into 10 cm/4 inch lengths. Onions, shallots and garlic can be roasted in their skins or peeled. The skins can be removed when they are cooked. Pumpkin when in season, marrow and squashes can also be included.

5. There is no need to bake vegetables in inches of oil. Simply roll them in a baking try in a little olive oil and add stock if they become too dry. Keep basting them and remove any that you feel are cooking too quickly and replace to reheat just before serving.

6. Place in a preheated oven at 200°C/400°F/gas mark 6. Reduce the heat to 180°C/350°F/gas mark 4 for about 1 hour or until the vegetables are browned and tender.

STIR-FRIED VEGETABLES

You can use all or some of the suggested vegetables and others of your choosing.

Metric/Imperial		American
1	carrot	1
1	parsnip	1
slice	swede	slice
½	red pepper	½
½	green pepper	½
½	leek (or 1 onion or small bunch of spring onions)	½
handful	French beans	handful
	olive oil	
handful	mange tout	handful
2	garlic cloves, finely sliced	2
2 small	courgettes, cut into 7cm/3 inch strips	2 small
¼ small	cabbage, finely shredded	¼ small
1	fresh ginger root (about the size of a thumb) finely sliced or grated (optional)	1
½	fresh chilli (about the size of a pea pod, or bigger if you like it hot), sliced	½

1. Scrub and trim the root vegetables, wash and seed the peppers.

2. Cut the leek into 10cm/4 inch lengths (wash carefully, they can be gritty), then cut lengthways into 1cm/½ inch strips. Finely slice the onions.
3. Top and tail the beans and slice down the middle. The mange tout can be added whole.
4. Cover the bottom of a large frying pan with olive oil and heat (but not until smoking point), stir in vegetables and keep on medium heat.
5. Cover with a lid and shake or stir periodically until the vegetables are how you like them.

STOCK-'FRIED' VEGETABLES

This is a quick, low-calorie, tasty way of caramelizing vegetables. Use any vegetables of your choice, as for stir-frying.

Metric/Imperial		American
	vegetables of your choice	
2 tsp	vegetable stock powder or	2 tsp
	½ stock cube or ½ pint/	
	300ml/1¼ cups homemade	
	stock	

1. Boil about 1cm/½ inch of water in a large frying pan over a high heat.
2. Add the vegetables and sprinkle with the vegetable stock powder. Stir until the stock evaporates and begans to stick to the pan. The vegetables should be beginning to brown now.
3. Lower the heat, add a little water and with a wooden spoon loosen the sediment from the bottom of the pan, and stir the vegetables. By now the liquor should be a dark golden colour.
4. Cover with lid and allow the vegetables to absorb stock.

IDEAS FOR COMBINING VEGETABLES

Be inventive and mix different tastes.

1. Try pink parsnips! Add peeled, diced, raw beetroot to diced parsnips in equal quantities and cook together until tender. Drain, add a little oil and a handful of finely chopped fresh parsley. Serve hot.
2. Add a cupful of cooked butter beans (canned are fine) when a cauliflower is almost cooked. Serve hot with vinaigrette dressing and lots of chopped fresh chives or spring onions.
3. Combine mashed potato and cooked spinach, add a tablespoon of yogurt, sieved cottage cheese (better still single cream) and some black pepper.
4. Remove the discoloured part of the stem, quarter, wash and dry gem lettuce or wedges of iceberg lettuce, add a large handful of washed, topped and tailed mange tout. Roll them around in a large knob of butter in a frying pan for about 3 minutes. Serve hot – buttery and crunchy.
5. Mix and mash: potato, carrot, parsnip and swede with a knob of butter or a tablespoon of yogurt. You could include celeriac for a different flavour. It is the root of a type of celery. It looks like a small, light brown, rather gnarled swede. The texture is similar and it has a mild celery flavour. Treat it as you would swede. It is delicious raw and gives a good flavour when added grated to soups.

CARROTS, PEPPERS AND FRENCH BEANS WITH GINGER GLAZE

Metric/Imperial		American
piece	fresh ginger root (about the size of a large thumb) or 1 tsp dried ginger	piece
225ml/8fl oz	water	1 cup
½	lemon, juice of	½
1 tsp	vegetable stock powder (or a little sea salt)	1 tsp
2	carrots	2
1 large	red pepper	1 large
175g/6oz	fresh or frozen French beans	1½ cups
1 tsp	arrowroot or cornflour	1 tsp

1. To make the glaze, peel and grate the ginger, then simmer in the water, lemon juice and a stock or a good pinch of salt for 20 minutes.
2. Scrub and top the carrots, slice lengthways to about the diameter of the beans.
3. Trim around the stalk of pepper. Pull and twist the stalk and most of the seeds should come out with the top. Wash out the rest under running water. Cut in half lengthways then into strips about the diameter of the beans.
4. Steam or water 'fry' the vegetables (keep in rows). Being finely cut they will cook quickly. Do not over-cook.

5. Arrange the vegetables in a row on a warmed oval serving dish and keep warm.
6. Mix the arrowroot with a little cold water. Add to the glaze and simmer, stirring, until it thickens and clears.
7. Strain into a warm jug and pour down the centre of the row of vegetables.

BROCCOLI WITH CRUNCHY TOPPING

You should be eating as many green vegetables as you can. Broccoli is tasty simply steamed or boiled in the minimum of water and served with olive oil or a knob of butter. It hardly needs embellishment but you might enjoy this for a change.

Metric/Imperial		American
450g/1 lb	broccoli	1 lb
2 tbsp	cottage cheese	2 tbsp
2 tbsp	yogurt	2 tbsp
100g/4oz	cooked millet, buckwheat or couscous	½ cup
100g/4oz	ground hazelnuts sesame seeds	1 cup

1. Wash and break the broccoli into manageable pieces. Discard discoloured leaves and woody part of the stem. 'Fan' remaining stem (slit with a sharp knife). This equalizes the cooking time of the florets and the stems. The stems are much tougher.
2. Steam for about 7 minutes, or boil for about 5 minutes. It does not take long to cook. As soon as the stalk is tender place in a warm ovenproof dish.
3. Sieve the cottage cheese and pour over the broccoli.
4. Top with millet mixed with the hazelnuts, cottage cheese and yogurt, sprinkle with sesame seeds and place under a preheated medium grill for about 3 minutes.

CAULIFLOWER WITH ONION SAUCE

This does not have the appeal of cauliflower cheese but it is a tasty second best.

Metric/Imperial		American
1	cauliflower	1
	sea salt	
1 large	onion	1 large
1 tsp	white mustard or	1 tsp
	celery seeds (optional)	
1 tsp	olive oil	1 tsp
½	French onion stock cube	½
	(or 1 tsp vegetable or	
	onion stock powder)	
1 tbsp	arrowroot, cornflour or	1 tbsp
	substitute	
300ml/½ pint	milk (or substitute)	1⅓ cups
	freshly grated nutmeg	
	(optional)	

1. Wash and divide the cauliflower into florets, keep on the leaves. Finely chop the stalks.
2. Either steam or cook in a minimum of water, adding a little salt towards the end of cooking.
3. Peel and dice the onion. If you weep at the thought of preparing onions, do them underwater. It spares your tears. Peel and top and tail in a bowl of tepid water. Discard the peelings and change the water. Cut the onion in half and hold the flat side on the bottom of the bowl. Dice, strain and pat dry on kitchen paper.

4. Fry the seeds in the oil, add the onion and fry over a low heat until tender and pale golden.
5. With a wooden spoon stir in the stock and cornflour. Cook gently for about 1 minute, stirring all the time. If it becomes too dry add a little milk or substitute. Add the remaining milk slowly, stirring constantly.
6. Place the cauliflower in a warmed serving dish or on warmed plates and pour over the sauce. Grate a little nutmeg on top if you like it.

Variation:

For a lower calorie, fat and milk-free onion glaze:
Simmer the onions, seeds and stock for 15 minutes in 225ml/8fl.oz water. Blend 1½ tsp of arrowroot or cornflour with a little cold water and stir into the onions. Simmer for 2 minutes then pour over the cauliflower.

LEEK AND POTATO CAKES

Metric/Imperial		American
450g/1 lb	potatoes, scrubbed and cooked in salted water	1 lb
knob	butter or margarine (or 2 tsp oil)	knob
1 small	leek (or ½ large leek, including green), cut lengthways flour (or substitute), to dust oil, for frying	1 small

1. Top and tail the leek and split lengthways. Place the flat surface on a board and make several more lengthways slits.
2. Cut across the length then put the finely chopped leeks into a bowl of water. Wash thoroughly, strain and pat dry with kitchen paper or a teacloth.
3. Drain the potatoes and mash with the butter, margarine or oil.
4. Mix in the leeks with a fork. With floured hands form the mixture into rounds about 2cm/¾ inch thick and 7.5cm/3 inches in diameter.
5. Heat a little oil in a frying pan until hot, add the potato cakes, reduce the heat and cover with a lid or baking sheet (the steam is necessary to cook the leeks). Allow about 5 minutes each side.

Variation:

If you would rather grill the potato cakes, brush with oil
and cook under a low grill for about 10 minutes each side.

GOLDEN POTATO CAKE

Metric/Imperial		American
700g/1½ lb	potatoes	1½ lb
2 tbsp	oil, plus extra for the onion	2 tbsp
15g/½oz	butter	1 tbsp
½ tsp	salt	½ tsp
1	onion, finely chopped	1

1. Scrub the potatoes and boil in salted water for 10 minutes.
2. Drain and cover with cold water. When cool enough to handle, grate the flesh.
3. Gently fry the onion until pale golden colour and remove from pan. Pieces of onion left in the pan will burn – make sure only the flavoured oil is left.
4. Heat half the oil and butter in the frying pan and add half the potato.
5. Add the onion and make a 'sandwich' with the rest of the potato – pressing into a firm cake. Cook over a low heat for about 10 minutes, lifting a corner at times to check it is not becoming too brown.
6. Place a baking sheet or pyrex plate over the pan, and turn the pan so that the uncooked side is uppermost.
7. Heat the remaining oil and butter and slide the potato cake back into the pan to cook the other side.
8. Cook for a further 8–10 minutes then slide onto a warmed plate.

Variations:

You can add a handful of the herb of your choice, or 2 rashers of chopped fried bacon and 2 cloves of garlic. Or substitute spring onion or leek for the onion, or fry half a finely chopped red pepper with the onion.

CRISP TOMATO COURGETTES

Boiled or steamed courgettes can be rather bland. Here is a way to liven them up.

Metric/Imperial		American
4	courgettes	4
1 tbsp	flour (or substitute)	1 tbsp
2 tbsp	tomato purée	2 tbsp
2 tbsp	oil, to fry	2 tbsp

1. Wash the courgettes, top and tail, and dry thoroughly. Cut in half lengthways then across the middle. Roll in the flour then in the tomato purée.
2. Heat the oil in a frying pan. Cook the courgettes until crisp on the outside and as crunchy or as soft as you like them in the middle. You will need to keep turning them.

Note:

You could use the tomato sauce on page 109, puréed.

BAKED SWEET POTATO
WITH COTTAGE CHEESE AND CHIVES

Sweet potatoes (yams) do not belong to the potato family (nightshades) and are therefore safe for those who are intolerant to potatoes. Their skins are dark red and they are shaped like flatter, elongated potatoes. They can be used in the same way as potatoes and don't take quite as long to cook. This is particularly noticeable when baking.

If you can't find smooth cottage cheese, simply rub the cheese through a sieve with a tablespoon of yogurt, or use a soft goat's cheese.

Metric/Imperial		American
2	sweet potatoes	2
4 tbsp	smooth cottage cheese	4 tbsp
large handful	fresh chives or spring onions, chopped	large handful

1. Scrub and prick the sweet potatoes, and bake in a preheated oven at 200°C/400°F/gas mark 6 for about 40 minutes, depending on size.
2. Combine the cheese and chives. Make a lengthways slit in the potatoes and fill with the cheese and chive mixture.

Variation:

Some people find yams very sweet and like to add a squeeze of lemon juice to the cottage cheese, or have them with sour cream.

SAVOY CABBAGE AND SEAWEED

This is a lot more appetising than it sounds and abounds
with minerals and trace elements. It has a strong 'green'
taste that goes well with fish, egg or bean dishes.

Metric/Imperial		American
25g/1oz	dried seaweed (see page 21)	2 tbsp
700g/1½ lb	spring cabbage (spring greens)	1½ lb
small bunch	spring onions	small bunch
1 tsp	vegetable or onion stock powder (or a little sea salt)	1 tsp

1. Soak the seaweed in cold water while preparing the
   cabbage.
2. Shred and wash the cabbage and chop all but the
   discoloured end of the stalk finely.
3. Top and tail the spring onions, wash, split lengthways,
   then cut into 3.
4. Roll the seaweed into a cigar shape and cut into
   5mm/¼ inch strips with scissors.
5. Heat 5mm/¼ inch of water in a frying pan or large
   saucepan. Add the vegetables, and sprinkle with the
   stock or seasoning. Reduce the heat, cover and cook,
   stirring occasionally, until the vegetables are to your
   liking. Because they are shredded they will be ready in
   about 5 minutes.

BRUSSELS SPROUTS WITH
CHESTNUT PURÉE SAUCE

Children seem to despise Brussels sprouts. Their reputation is not wholly unjustified because they are so often overcooked – boiled to death in gallons of water. They can be shredded and used in green salads or stir-fries, or halved and boiled for 2–3 minutes, then rolled around in a covered frying pan over a low heat. They don't need to be fried so you will need only a small amount of butter. To this you could add either a crushed clove of garlic, or a teaspoonful of fennel seeds, caraway or cumin seeds.

Metric/Imperial		American
100g/4oz	cooked chestnuts (see below)	½ cup
4 tbsp	milk (or substitute)	4 tbsp
knob	butter	knob
350g/12oz	Brussels sprouts	¾ lb

1. To cook fresh chestnuts (lovely but a bit of a hassle to do), cover with cold water and boil in their skins for 1–1½ hours. Cool, peel and remove any fibrous pieces in the centre.
2. To cook dried chestnuts (easier), soak overnight then boil for 45 minutes–1 hour. (You can also buy cans of prepared chestnut sauce!)
3. Heat the chestnuts in the milk. Add the butter and mash, blend or rub through a sieve. Keep warm.

4. Remove any discoloured leaves from the sprouts, trim
    the stalks and wash. If they are large, halve them. Put
    into boiling water with a little sea salt for about 4–7
    minutes. Do not overcook. Serve immediately topped
    with the sauce.

HARD WHITE CABBAGE WITH APPLES

Some dessert apples 'fall', that is they go soft like cooking apples but it does not matter for this recipe if they stay crunchy.

Metric/Imperial		American
½	hard white cabbage	½
1	cooking apple	1
2	dessert apples	2
½	lemon, juice of	½
½ tsp	salt	½ tsp

1. Shred the cabbage, and chop all but the woody stalk finely. Wash and drain.
2. Peel the apples, core and slice thinly.
3. Boil 1cm/½ inch of water in a large frying pan (can be done in a saucepan but needs stirring more frequently). Add the cabbage, apples and lemon juice.
4. Reduce the heat, cover and stir after about 3 minutes. When the cabbage is almost tender add the salt. Cooks in about 6 minutes.
5. Serve with pork or ham dishes.

AUBERGINE CURRY

Metric/Imperial		American
1	aubergine	1
	salt	
1 small	onion, chopped	1 small
2	garlic cloves, chopped	2
1 small	fresh green chilli, chopped	1 small
2 tbsp	oil	2 tbsp
1 tsp	turmeric	1 tsp
¼ tsp	ground black pepper	¼ tsp
½ tsp	black mustard seeds	½ tsp
225g/8oz	tomatoes, or canned (citric acid-free) tomatoes, chopped	1 cup
bunch	fresh coriander, chopped	bunch

1. Slice the aubergines into 1cm/½ inch thick pieces. Sprinkle with salt and leave for 30 minutes (this removes the bitter taste). Rinse, dry and quarter.
2. Fry the onion, garlic and chilli for 5 minutes until golden brown.
3. Add the turmeric, pepper and mustard seeds. Stir until the seeds begin to pop. Add aubergines and fry for 5 minutes.
4. Add the tomatoes and cook for 15–20 minutes, uncovered, to reduce the liquid.
5. Add the coriander and stir for 30 seconds.
6. Serve with brown rice and plain yogurt.

DRY MILD POTATO
AND CARROT CURRY

Metric/Imperial		American
2 tsp	cumin seeds	2 tsp
225g/8oz	carrots, diced	1⅓ cups
225g/8oz	potatoes, diced	1⅓ cups
¼–½ tsp	chilli powder	¼–½ tsp
½ tsp	turmeric	½ tsp
1 tsp	ground coriander	1 tsp
125ml/4fl oz	water	½ cup
	salt, to taste	
1–2 tbsp	oil	1–2 tbsp

1. Heat the oil and fry the cumin seeds until they crackle.
2. Add the diced vegetables and fry for 5–6 minutes.
3. Add the chilli, turmeric and coriander, and fry for 1 minute.
4. Add the water, cover and cook for 5–7 minutes until the vegetables are tender and the mixture is dry.
5. Serve with main dishes or rice and plain yogurt.

STUFFED ONIONS

Metric/Imperial		American
4	onions	4
2	potatoes, scrubbed and roughly chopped	2
2 tsp	dried sage	2 tsp
knob	butter	knob
large pinch	salt	large pinch
	oil, for brushing	

1. Peel the onions and boil whole with the potatoes for 15 minutes.
2. Lift out the onions with a slotted spoon and leave until cool enough to handle.
3. Drain the potatoes and return to the pan. Add the sage, butter and salt, and mash.
4. Cut the top third from the onions and lift out the middles with a fork (a gentle squeeze from the bottom might help), leaving only a shell of 2 or 3 outer layers.
5. Finely chop the saved onion and add to the mashed potato.
6. Fill the shells with the mixture and brush with oil.
7. Place on a baking sheet on a low shelf in a preheated oven at 220°C/425°F/gas mark 7, reducing the heat immediately to 180°C/350°F/gas mark 4, and bake for 20 minutes.

Variations:

Reconstitute a packet of sage and onion stuffing with boiling water (don't worry about this – you will be using very few convenience foods) and mix in the saved onion.

If you are restricting carbohydrate use chopped cooked spinach instead of potato, and simply mash with the sage and butter.

6

Main Meals

MEAT DOES NOT encourage fungal growth unless, as mentioned, it is contaminated with antibiotics or steroids. Organic meat is 'clean' but unfortuately not widely available and can be expensive. Some butchers can tell you the source of their meat and give information of how it is reared. If you enjoy meat, eat it regularly. It is high in zinc, iron and many other nutrients and because it is digested slowly keeps the blood sugar levels stable and prevents sugar cravings. If you have digestive troubles do not eat meat with potatoes. Lamb and rabbit do not contain antibiotics or steroids. The candida diet is an eating plan to correct a medical condition. Some vegetarians are temporarily willing to include meat if they are very depleted. The body needs protein for repairing cells and boosting the immune system. Meat is a first class protein.

YOGURT BAKED CHICKEN

Metric/Imperial		American
4	chicken thighs or breasts, skinned and trimmed	4
2	garlic cloves, crushed or finely chopped	2
1 tbsp	dried (or 2 tbsp chopped fresh) mint	1 tbsp
½ tsp	salt	½ tsp
6 tbsp	plain yogurt	6 tbsp

1. Make 2 deep cuts across the chicken joints and place on an oiled baking tray.
2. Combine the garlic, mint, salt and yogurt. Spoon over the chicken and leave for at least 2 hours, preferably overnight.
3. Bake in a preheated oven at 200°C/400°F/gas mark 6 for 35 minutes.
4. Serve with broccoli or spring greens, peas and new potatoes.

CARAWAY CABBAGE WITH CHICKEN

This dish is designed to erase all memories of school dinner cabbage and show what a remarkably interesting vegetable the humble cabbage can be.

Metric/Imperial		*American*
4 tsp	olive oil (or oil of your choice)	4 tsp
4 pieces	chicken (eg breasts, legs, thighs), skinned	4 pieces
½	white cabbage, stalk included, shredded	½
2 tsp	caraway or cumin seeds	2 tsp
½	vegetable stock cube (or 1 tsp stock powder)	½
150ml/¼ pint	water	⅔ cup

1. In a large frying pan using hot (but not smoking) oil, fry the chicken until golden brown – about 10 minutes each side.
2. Add the shredded cabbage. Sprinkle with caraway seeds and stock powder or press the stock cube onto the base of the pan and mix with the juices from chicken.
3. Keep the heat high and stir until the bottom of the pan begins to colour. Don't worry if it looks dark, the liquor from this dish looks almost the colour of soy sauce.

4. Add the water, a little at a time, using a wooden spoon to blend the caramelized juices from the bottom of the pan.
5. Cover and cook over a low heat, stirring occasionally, until the chicken is tender.

CURRIED BROWN RICE

Metric/Imperial		American
1 tsp	turmeric	1 tsp
1 tsp	curry powder	1 tsp
4	cardamom pods	4
2	cloves	2
¼	stick cinnamon (or ½ tsp cinnamon powder)	¼
2 tbsp	olive oil	2 tbsp
1	onion, finely chopped	1
2	garlic cloves, finely chopped or crushed	2
225g/8oz	brown rice	1 cup
475ml/16fl oz	chicken or vegetable stock	2 cups
1 tsp	salt	1 tsp

1. Gently fry the spices in the oil for about 1 minute.
2. Add the onion and garlic and fry until golden.
3. Add the rice and fry until it has taken on the colour of the spices.
4. Add the stock and salt and bring to boil, then transfer to a saucepan if the frying pan does not have a close-fitting lid.
5. Cover and cook over a gentle heat until the stock is absorbed and the rice is cooked. The time will depend on the rice, usually 35–45 minutes. Check periodically to see if a little water is needed, but take care not to flood it or it will be soggy.

6. Can be kept warm in a casserole covered with a damp tea cloth, or placed in a steamer on a low heat.

Variations:

Add any or all of the following – 2 tbsp cooked peas, 4 tbsp cooked shrimps, 3 tbsp finely chopped spring onions, 2 tbsp toasted cashew nuts or almonds, 1 dessert-spoon toasted cumin seeds.

LAMB AND MINT CAKES

Minced lamb can be bought prepacked in some super-markets, or ask for stewing lamb from your butcher who will mince it for you.

Metric/Imperial		American
1 small	onion	1 small
1	carrot	1
1	potato	1
225g/8oz	minced lamb	½ lb
1 tsp	salt	1 tsp
2 tsp	dried mint (or handful of fresh mint), finely chopped, flour (or substitute), for dusting oil, for frying	2 tsp

1. Peel and grate the onion.
2. Scrub the carrot and potato and grate (squeeze the water out of the grated potato).
3. Place all the ingredients in a bowl and mix thoroughly with a knife. Press the mixture firmly together.
4. Divide into balls, dust with flour and press into patties about 2cm/¾ inch thick and 7.5cm/3 inches in diameter.
5. Fry on one side in a little hot oil over medium heat for 5 minutes, then lower the heat and cook for a further 10 minutes.

6. Lift out the patties and raise the temperature of the oil. Return them to the pan and fry the other side in the same way.

LAMB AND MINT SHEPHERD'S PIE

Metric/Imperial		American
225g/8oz	minced lamb	½ lb
1	onion, finely chopped	1
1	carrot, scrubbed and diced	1
1	stock cube (lamb, chicken or vegetable) or 2 rounded tsp vegetable stock powder or 1 tsp salt	1
2 tsp	dried mint (or large handful of fresh mint), chopped	2 tsp
	water, to cover	
2 tsp	flour (or substitute), blended with a little cold water (or 1 small potato, grated)	2 tsp
450g/1lb	potatoes, cooked, drained and mashed with knob of butter and 2 tbsp milk or substitute	1 lb

1. Gently fry the meat, onion and carrot for about 5 minutes.
2. Transfer the mixture to a saucepan, add the stock cube, peas and mint and enough water to cover. Simmer, covered, for 30 minutes.
3. Thicken with the flour mixture or grated potato.
4. Transfer to a pie dish and top with the mashed potato. Smooth the top with a fork and brush with oil or add a few knobs of butter and a little black pepper if liked.

5. Bake under a moderate grill until the topping is crisp.

Note:

If you are on a low fat diet, cool the meat mixture and refrigerate for a couple of hours. The fat will then lift off easily. Also mash the potatoes with low fat plain yogurt.

HARICOT BEANS IN TOMATO SAUCE

Metric/Imperial		American
175g/6oz	haricot beans	¾ cup
piece	dried kombu (sea vegetable) (optional)	piece
2 tsp	vegetable stock powder (or 1 stock cube or ½ tsp salt)	2 tsp

Tomato sauce

2 tbsp	oil	2 tbsp
450g/1lb	ripe tomatoes	1 lb
1 small	onion, finely chopped	1 small
2	garlic cloves, crushed	2
½	red pepper (optional), finely chopped	½
1 tsp	honey or sugar (optional)	1 tsp

1. If the beans have been soaking overnight, drain, put in saucepan and cover with cold water.
2. Bring to the boil and simmer until tender (about 1¼–1½ hours). Add the vegetable stock powder, cube or salt near the end of the cooking time.
3. If the beans have not been soaked overnight, bring to the boil and cook for 3 minutes, remove from the heat, keep covered and leave to stand for 1 hour. Drain, cover with fresh water and cook as above.

4. To make the tomato sauce, fry the ingredients slowly in the oil for 30 minutes, covered, giving an occasional stir. It should now be like a purée.
5. Drain the beans and combine with the sauce. Cook gently together for 10 minutes to allow the beans to absorb the tomato flavour. If there is not enough liquid, add stock or tomato juice.

LEEK AND BROCCOLI BAKE

Metric/Imperial		American
1	leek	1
225g/8oz	broccoli	½ lb
½ tsp	salt	½ tsp
600ml/1 pint	soya milk (or substitute)	2½ cups
2	eggs, beaten and seasoned	2

1. Chop the leek finely (including the green part), wash and drain.
2. Break the broccoli into florets, and cut the stem into 1cm/½ inch pieces. Discard only the woody pieces of stalk.
3. Cover the vegetables with water, bring to the boil and simmer for 5 minutes, adding salt in the last minute. Drain and put in a pie dish.
4. Warm the milk in a pan and pour onto the eggs. Return the liquid to the pan and heat until it thickens, stirring constantly. Do not allow to boil.
5. Pour the liquid over the vegetables, and bake in a preheated oven at 170°C/325°F/gas mark 3 for 15–20 minutes until set.

QUICK VEGETABLE HOT POT

Any combination of vegetables can be used for this. You could also add a layer of tomato sauce (page 109) before adding the sliced potato.

Metric/Imperial		American
4	potatoes	4
1	leek, chopped	1
1 large	carrot, chopped	1 large
¼	swede, chopped	¼
2	tomatoes, chopped	2
1	vegetable stock cube (or 1 tsp vegetable stock)	1
100g/4oz	canned low-sugar baked beans	½ cup
	oil, for brushing	
	sesame or sunflower seeds, for sprinkling	

1. Cut 3 of the potatoes in half, boil until tender, drain and set aside.
2. Place all the vegetables, except the 4 potatoes, in a saucepan. Add the stock cube and enough water to come about half way up the vegetables.
3. Grate the whole uncooked potato and add to the pan. Bring to the boil, cover and simmer until tender.
4. Add the baked beans and stir through until heated, then transfer to an ovenproof dish.

5. Slice the cooked potatoes and arrange on top of the vegetable mixture. Brush with oil, sprinkle with sesame seeds and brown under a preheated medium grill until crisp and golden.

ROAST LEG OF LAMB
WITH GARLIC, THYME AND MINT

A fillet (thick slice of leg) or half a shoulder of lamb could also be used. The rich herb and garlic flavour penetrates the meat. It goes well with simple steamed vegetables, particularly broccoli, cauliflower and carrots. Tiny new potatoes are a treat with this but not if you have digestive problems.

Metric/Imperial		American
1 small	leg of lamb	1 small
6	garlic cloves	6
1 tbsp	olive oil	1 tbsp
1 tbsp	dried mint	1 tbsp
1 tbsp	dried thyme	1 tbsp

1. Wash and dry the joint and trim off excess fat. With a sharp pointed knife make 9 deep cuts on each side of the joint.
2. Peel and slice the garlic lengthways into 3 slivers. Slide these into the slits in the joint.
3. Brush the joint with the oil and sprinkle both sides with the herbs and salt.
4. Roast in a preheated oven at 200°C/400°F/gas mark 6 for 20 minutes.

5. Reduce the heat to 180°C/350°F/gas mark 4 for a further 40 minutes. At this stage it should be a little rare in the middle. Test it by piercing with a sharp knife at the thickest part of the joint. If the juices run too red for you, cook for another 20 minutes.

SPLIT PEAS WITH BROWN RICE

This has a nutty, slightly sweet flavour. It makes a sustaining main dish, accompanied by spinach or spring greens. Leftovers can be made into tasty Vegeburgers (see opposite).

Metric/Imperial		American
175g/6oz	split peas	1 cup
2 heaped tsp	stock power (or 2 stock cubes or 1 tsp salt)	2 heaped tsp
1.25 litres/ 2¼ pints	water	6 cups
175g/6oz	brown rice, washed	¾ cup

1. Wash the split peas and discard any stones.
2. Simmer in the stock and water for 15 minutes.
3. Add the rice and simmer for a further 40–45 minutes.

VEGEBURGERS

Metric/Imperial		American
175g/6oz	cold Split Peas with Brown Rice (see opposite)	¾ cup
1	small carrot, finely chopped or grated	1
4	spring onions, 4 shallots or 1 small onion, finely chopped	4
large handful	fresh parsley, chopped	large handful
1 tbsp	sesame seeds, flour or rice flour, for dusting oil, for frying	1 tbsp

1. Combine the ingredients and shape into rounds about 2cm/¾ inch thick. Dust with sesame seeds or flour.
2. Fry gently on each side for 7–10 minutes.

BUCKWHEAT PANCAKES

These can be eaten with a savoury filling such as tuna and mayonnaise, spinach and potatoes or for breakfast with stewed fruit and yogurt or low sugar marmalade.

Metric/Imperial		American
50g/2oz	buckwheat flour	½ cup
50g/2oz	cornmeal or fine oatmeal	½ cup
½ tsp	baking powder	½ tsp
½ tsp	bicarbonate of soda	½ tsp
1	egg, beaten	1
400ml/12fl oz	buttermilk (or substitute)	1½ cups
2 tbsp	melted butter or oil	2 tbsp
	oil, for frying	

1. Mix the dry ingredients in a bowl.
2. Combine the egg, buttermilk or substitute, and melted butter or oil.
3. Make a batter by adding the liquid to the dry ingredients, a little at a time.
4. Lightly oil a heavy frying pan and slowly heat it.
5. Fry 2 tbsp of the batter at a time in the pan. When bubbles appear on the surface and the edge looks dry, turn and cook the other side.
6. Add a little water if the batter becomes too thick.

Variation:

Replace the buttermilk with half and half water and soya milk (or cow's milk) or plain yogurt.

GRILLED HERRING IN OATMEAL

Fatty fish such as herring and mackerel are a very useful part of the anticandida diet. As well as being sustaining, they are rich in essential oils which are necessary for a healthy immune system, and they keep the blood sugar levels stable. Cheaper than white fish, they are quick and simple to prepare. Herrings are easier to digest if you don't eat carbohydrate with them.

Metric/Imperial		American
4	herring fillets	4
	oil, for brushing	
2 tbsp	fine oatmeal	2 tbsp

1. Wash the fillets thoroughly to remove any traces of blood. Pat dry with kitchen paper and brush with a little oil.
2. Sprinkle the oatmeal onto a plate, and press the flesh side onto this. It is not necessary to oatmeal the skin side as they will not need turning.
3. Cook under a preheated hot grill until they are crisp and golden.
4. Serve with salad or a green vegetable.

GRILLED MACKEREL WITH
LEMON YOGURT SAUCE

Metric/Imperial		American
2	mackerel fillets	2
4 tbsp	plain yogurt	4 tbsp
½	lemon, juice of	½
1 tsp	grated lemon zest	1 tsp

1. Wash the fillets and pat dry with kitchen paper. Combine the yogurt and lemon.
2. Place the fish under a preheated hot grill for 5 minutes, then spread with yogurt and lemon mixture.
3. Lower the heat and grill for a further 5–7 minutes.
4. Serve with salad, broccoli or green beans.

HAKE IN DILL MARINADE

Hake is a firm-textured fish with a good flavour.

Metric/Imperial		American
2	hake steaks	2
	oil, for frying (optional)	

Marinade

3 tbsp	olive oil	3 tbsp
squeeze	lemon juice	squeeze
¼ tsp	salt	¼ tsp
2 tbsp	finely chopped fresh dill	2 tbsp
	(or 1 tsp dill seeds, crushed)	

1. Combine the marinade ingredients.
2. Wash and dry the hake steaks, and place in the marinade for at least 8 hours. Turn several times.
3. Either fry slowly for about 7 minutes each side, or place in 1cm/½ inch of boiling water in a small frying pan, reduce the heat, cover and simmer for about 30 minutes. Do not turn. The water will reduce during cooking and steam the fish which should be tender and moist.

GRILLED SALMON WITH FENNEL SAUCE

Grilled salmon is a quick tasty meal and stands well with just a squeeze of lemon served with a green salad. If you want a change try it with fennel. You can add it to the salad or put it in a yogurt or mayonnaise dressing. It is crisp and tender and adds a delicate aniseed flavour.

Metric/Imperial		*American*
1 bulb	fennel (or 1 tbsp fennel seeds)	1 bulb
	butter, for frying and grilling	
	plain yogurt, for the sauce	
2	salmon steaks	2

1. To make the sauce, top and tail the fresh fennel and chop finely. Fry gently in a little butter or oil in a covered pan until tender.
2. Rub through a sieve or liquidize, season and add 2 tbsp yogurt. Return to the pan to keep warm.
3. If using fennel seeds, fry gently in a little butter or oil until the colour changes. Reduce the heat, season and stir in 3 tbsp yogurt.
4. Wash and dry the salmon. Top with a knob of butter and grill on one side under a moderate heat for 3–5 minutes depending on thickness.
5. Turn, add a knob of butter and grill until golden brown.
6. Transfer to heated serving plates and serve with the sauce and green vegetables.

Candida Albicans

STIR-FRY PORK FILLET
WITH GREEN PEPPERS

Pork fillet is a lean boneless cut which looks like a flat-tened large sausage. It is a little more expensive than other cuts of pork but worth it for this dish. Pieces of pork sliced off the leg can be used, but it may not be quite so tender and does have a border of fat.

Metric/Imperial		*American*
255g/8oz	pork fillet	½ lb
1	green pepper	1
1	leek, finely sliced	1
100g/4oz	beansprouts (optional)	2 cups
	oil, for frying	

1. Wash and dry the pork and cut into 5cm x 1cm/2 inch x ½ inch strips.
2. Cut the pepper into 2.5cm x 1cm/1 inch x ½ inch pieces.
3. Fry the pork quickly in a little hot oil for 2 minutes then remove from the pan.
4. Fry the sliced leek until tender, then add the pepper pieces.
5. Return the pork to the pan and stir until tender. Don't overcook. The pepper pieces need to retain some of their texture.

FLUFFY SPINACH OMELETTE

Metric/Imperial		American
4	eggs, separated	4
2 tbsp	cold water	2 tbsp
225g/8oz	chopped cooked spinach (fresh or frozen)	1 cup
	salt	
	oil, for frying	

1. Whisk the egg whites until stiff.
2. Beat the yolks with the water and a good pinch of salt, then fold into the egg whites.
3. Heat the spinach, then strain, pressing onto the strainer with the back of a spoon to remove any liquid. Return to the pan, season and keep warm.
4. Heat a thin film of oil in a small frying pan (about 18cm/7 inches in diameter) to just below smoking point.
5. Add the egg mixture, reduce the heat to low, and cover.
6. Leave for 5 minutes then spoon the spinach over half the mixture. Turn half of the omelette over to cover the spinach. Cover and leave for a further 5 minutes or until the omelette is set.

SHRIMP-STUFFED PLAICE

Metric/Imperial		American
4 small or	fillets of plaice	4 small or
2 large		2 large
100g/4oz	cooked shrimps	½ cup
knob	butter	knob
2 tbsp	chopped fresh parsley	2 tbsp

1. Wash the plaice and remove any remnants of bone left at the head end. Dry.
2. Skin any grey-skinned fillets by lifting the flesh with a sharp knife at the tail and holding the skin. Pull the skin towards you and gently ease the flesh away from you with the knife.
3. Mash the shrimps with the butter, then add the parsley. Spoon the mixture onto the fillets and roll up from the head end. Secure with a cocktail stick, or pack tightly in a steamer so they don't unroll.
4. Steam for 10–15 minutes.
5. If you don't have a steamer you can put them between 2 plates over a saucepan of boiling water.

WHITING WITH BROAD BEANS
AND PARSLEY BUTTER

Whiting is an underrated fish. It is cheap, has a very good flavour and the texture is much firmer than cod. Look for large fillets.

Metric/Imperial		American
handful	parsley, finely chopped	handful
25g/1oz	butter	2 tbsp
2 large	fillets of whiting	2 large
	oil, for brushing	
225g/8oz	broad beans	1⅓ cups
50g/2oz	fresh sweetcorn (optional)	⅓ cup

1. Blend the parsley with the butter and divide the mixture into two.
2. Wash the whiting and remove any bones left at the head end. Dry, brush with oil and place on an oiled baking tray under a preheated medium grill until golden brown.
3. Boil the beans and corn together until tender, strain and serve topped with parsley butter on heated plates with the fish.

MRS JAMES'S CHICKEN

For a traditional Jamaican feel, serve with rice and peas and coleslaw.

Metric/Imperial		American
4	joints chicken, skinned	4
1 heaped tsp	curry powder	1 heaped tsp
½ tsp	ground allspice, thyme or oregano	½ tsp
1 tsp	black pepper	1 tsp
¼ tsp	salt	¼ tsp
1 large	onion, finely chopped	1 large
4	garlic cloves, crushed	4
2 tbsp	olive or sunflower oil	2 tbsp
½	red pepper, finely sliced	½

1. Rub the dry spices into the chicken, then press on the onion and garlic. Leave for 4 hours or overnight.
2. Heat the oil in a heavy casserole, dust the onion and garlic off the chicken and save. Brown the chicken in the oil. Add the onion and garlic and fry for 2 minutes.
3. Cover with water and simmer, covered, for 1 hour.
4. Add the red pepper and simmer for 30 minutes.

HELEN'S FAVOURITE DAHL

Metric/Imperial		American
Lentil mixture		
225g/8oz	red lentils, washed and soaked	1 cup
6	garlic cloves, crushed	6
2 tsp	grated fresh ginger root	2 tsp
1–2	dried red chillies, crumbled	1–2
½ tsp	paprika	½ tsp
½ tsp	turmeric	½ tsp
Spice mixture		
25g/1oz	butter	2 tbsp
½ tsp	paprika	½ tsp
1	onion, chopped	1
2 tsp	grated fresh ginger root	2 tsp
1	fresh green chilli, chopped	1
2 tsp	ground cumin	2 tsp
2 tsp	ground coriander	2 tsp
400g/14oz	canned tomatoes	2 cups
½ tsp	garam masala (optional)	½ tsp

1. Put the ingredients for the lentil mixture in a pan, cover with water and cook for 20–30 minutes until the lentils are soft.
2. Heat the butter, remove from the heat and add the paprika.

3. Return to the heat and add the onion, ginger and chilli. Fry for 5 minutes, then add the cumin and coriander and fry for 2 minutes.
4. Stir in the tomatoes.
5. Add this mixture to the pan of cooked lentils and stir well.
6. Just before serving, add the garam masala.
7. Serve with brown rice and plain yogurt. Can also be used cold as a dip for raw vegetables.

QUICK DAHL FOR BUSY PEOPLE (MILD)

Metric/Imperial		American
225g/8oz	red lentils	1 cup
2 tsp	curry powder	2 tsp
1 tsp	vegetable stock powder (or ¼ tsp salt)	1 tsp
2	cloves (optional)	2
2.5cm/1 inch	piece cinnamon stick (or ½ tsp ground cinnamon)	1 inch
6	cardamom pods	6

1. Put all the ingredients in a pan and cover with about 2.5cm/1 inch of water.
2. Boil quickly (adding more water if necessary), for about 25 minutes or until the lentils have formed a purée.
3. Serve with Chapatis (page 137), brown rice or vegetables.

QUICK CHICK PEA CURRY

Metric/Imperial		American
1	potato, diced	1
50g/2oz	fresh or frozen peas	⅓ cup
1 small	onion, chopped	1 small
2	garlic cloves, chopped	2
1 heaped tsp	curry powder	1 heaped tsp
	oil for frying	
400g/14oz	canned chick peas, drained	2 cups

1. Cook the potato and peas in salted water until tender. Drain.
2. Fry the onion, garlic and curry powder slowly for 3 minutes.
3. Add the chick peas, potatoes and peas. Heat through, adding a little water if necessary, but don't drown it. The dish should be quite dry.
4. Serve with finely sliced onions and tomatoes, or if you can take wheat and are not severely restricting carbohydrates, you can use this mixture as a filling for samosas (see next page).

SAMOSAS

Metric/Imperial		American
225g/8oz	wholemeal flour	2 cups
2 tbsp	oil, plus extra for deep frying	2 tbsp
	warm water, for mixing	

1. Mix the flour and oil with enough warm water to make a soft dough.
2. Chill for at least 2 hours.
3. Roll out thinly and cut into 10cm/4 inch squares. Spoon on the chick pea curry mixture. Make triangle shape and nip the edges.
4. Deep fry for about 3 minutes until golden brown.

7

Alternatives to Yeasted Bread

I F YOU DON'T have time to bake, rice cakes, rye crisp-breads, oatcakes and pumpernickel are widely available. Check that the brand you choose is yeast-free and if you are wheat intolerant, wheat-free. Buckwheat Pancakes (page 118) are also a good bread substitute.

OAT CAKES

Metric/Imperial		American
175g/6oz	fine oatmeal	1½ cup
½ tsp	salt	½ tsp
½ tsp	bicarbonate of soda	½ tsp
1 tbsp	oil or melted butter	1 tbsp
2 tsp	honey or 1 tsp fructose (fruit sugar)	2 tsp
60ml/2½fl oz	boiling water	¼ cup

1. Combine the dry ingredients in a mixing bowl.
2. Blend the oil or butter, honey and boiling water in another bowl.
3. Add the dry ingredients and knead until smooth.
4. Shape the mixture into a round and roll out very thinly to a diameter of about 25.5cm/10 inches.
5. Heat oven to 150°C/300°F/gas mark 2 for 35–40 minutes.

Variations:

Replace 50g/2oz of the oatmeal with the same quantity of either ground sesame seeds or ground sunflower seeds.

YEAST-FREE WHOLEMEAL LOAF

Metric/Imperial		American
225g/8oz	wholemeal flour	2 cups
1½ tbsp	olive oil	1½ tbsp
300ml/10fl oz	milk or buttermilk	1⅓ cups
1½ tsp	bicarbonate of soda	1½ tsp
2 tsp	honey	2 tsp

1. Combine the dry ingredients in a mixing bowl.
2. Whisk together the honey, oil and milk, and mix into the dry ingredients with a knife.
3. Knead into a dough, then roll out to a round, about 3cm/1¼ inches thick.
4. Place on an oiled baking sheet and cook in a preheated oven at 200°C/400°F/gas mark 6 for 30–35 minutes.

Variations:

Replace the milk with soya milk or half yogurt and half water.

STEVE'S WHEAT-FREE
YEAST-FREE BREAD

Metric/Imperial		American
2 tsp	honey (optional)	2 tsp
125ml/4fl oz	soya yogurt	½ cup
2 tbsp	sunflower oil	2 tbsp
1	egg, beaten until frothy	1
50g/2oz	maize meal	4 tbsp
40g/1½oz	gram flour (chick pea flour)	3 tbsp
65g/2½oz	barley flour	5 tbsp
½ tsp	salt	½ tsp
1½ tsp	bicarbonate of soda (or 2 tsp baking powder)	1½ tsp

1. Blend the honey with the yogurt, add the oil and beat into the egg.
2. Mix the dry ingredients and beat a little at a time into the liquid. It makes quite a thick batter. If you have a blender you can just throw in all the ingredients and whiz!
3. Pour the mixture into a greased loaf tin and bake at 200°C/400°F/gas mark 6 for 20–25 minutes.

CHAPATIS

Metric/Imperial		American
225g/8oz	fine wheatmeal flour	2 cups
1 tsp	salt	1 tsp
4 tsp	oil	4 tsp
225ml/8fl oz	tepid water	1 cup

1. Reserve 1 heaped tbsp of the flour and place the rest in a bowl with the salt. Make a well in the centre, and add the water and oil.
2. Knead for at least 10 minutes into a soft dough.
3. Put in a plastic bag and refrigerate for at least 1 hour, preferably overnight.
4. Cut the dough into 4 pieces, then make 3 balls from each piece.
5. Using the reserved flour, roll the balls out on a floured board until about 12.5cm/5 inches in diameter.
6. Heat a heavy frying pan, and cook the chapatis one at a time. Press the edges of the chapati to the pan with a folded tea towel to trap air.
7. Cook for 1 minute on each side.

Variations:

Add 3 crushed cloves of garlic to the flour.
Add 2 tsp cumin seeds to the flour.
Omit the salt and oil.

Further Reading

The British Medical Association Guide to Medicine and Drugs (for prescription and over-the-counter medications), Dorling Kindersley, 1989

Brostoff, Dr Jonathon and Gamlin, Linda. *Food Allergy and Intolerance*, Bloomsbury, 1989

Chaitow, Leon. *Candida Albicans: Could Yeast Be Your Problem?*, Thorsons, 1991

Crook, William G. MD. *The Yeast Connection* (Professional Books/Future Health, Inc., PO Box 3246, Jackson, Tennessee 38303–0846, USA)

Davies, Dr Stephen and Stewart, Dr Alan. *Nutritional Medicine*, Bloomsbury, 1989

Grant, Doris and Joice, Jean. *Food Combining for Health*, Thorsons, 1984

Kenton, Leslie and Susannah. *Raw Energy*, Century Arrow, 1984

Markarness, Dr Richard. *Not all in the Mind*, Thorsons, 1995

Patterson, Barbara. *The Allergy Connection*, Thorsons, 1995

Rippere, Vickey. *The Allergy Problem*, Thorsons, 1989

Trickett, Shirley. *Coping with Anxiety and Depression*, Sheldon Press, 1989 (see 'Other Causes of Nervous Illness)

Trickett, Shirley. *Coping with Candida*, Sheldon Press, 1994

Trickett, Shirley. *Coping Successfully with Panic Attacks*, Sheldon Press, 1992. (see 'Sugar and Spice and all Things Nice')

Trickett, Shirley. *The Irritable Bowel and Diverticulosis*, Thorsons, 1990

Truss, C. Orion MDPO. *The Missing Diagnosis* (Box 26508), Birmingham, AL 35226)

Useful Addresses

IBS NETWORK
Run by IBS (Irritable Bowel Syndrome) sufferers for
IBS sufferers. It offers:
– quarterly newsletter Gut Reaction
– self help groups
– 'Can't wait' card
For further information send an sae to IBS Network, c/o
Centre for Human Nutrition, Northern General
Hospital, Sheffield, S5 7AU

Action Against Allergy
Amelia Hill
43 The Downs
London SW20
AAA (Action Against Allergy) provides an information
service on all aspects of allergy and allergy-related
illness, which is free to everyone. Supporting members
get a newsletter three times a year and a postal lending
library service. AAA can supply GPs with the names and
addresses of specialist allergy doctors. It also has a talk-

line network which puts sufferers in telephone touch with others through the NHS and itself initiates and supports research. Enclose sae (9 x 6 inches) for further information.

Institute of Allergy Therapists: short courses in the diagnosis and treatment of allergic conditions. The Institute maintains a Register of Practitioners and provides a referral service for the general public. Write to: Donald M Harrison, B A (Hons), B Sc, M R Pharm S, Institute of Allergy Therapists, Ffynnonwen, Llangwyryfon, Aberystwyth, Dyfed, SY23 4EY.

National Society for Research into Allergy
PO Box 45
Hinkley
Leicestershire LE10 1JY

British Holistic Medical Association
179 Gloucester Place
London NW1 6DX

Society for Environmental Therapy
3 Atherton Street
Ipswich
Suffolk IP4 2LD

National Institute of Medical Herbalists
PO Box 3, Winchester, SO22 6RB

Wholefood, Organically Grown Produce
24 Paddington Street
London W1M 4DR

New Nutrition
Woodlands
London Road
Battle
East Sussex TN33 0LP
Tel 01424 774103
Experienced nutritional advice for Irritable Bowel and
other colon problems: health letter service, telephone and
personal consultations, send sae for details.

BioCare Limited
54 Northfield Road
Norton
Birmingham B30 1JH
Tel 0121 433 3727
Wide range of nutritional supplements for Candida
control and allergies including: Mycropryl – slow release
Caprylic Acid, Cystoplex – cranberry juice capsules,
Butyric Acid Complex – food allergies. BioCare is the
only UK company in the practitioner market that manu-
factures its own range of Probiotics in its own facilities.
BioCare's Bio-Acidophilus is the only Probiotic on the
UK market derived from a research grant from the
British Government Department of Trade and Industry.

Family Health & Nutrition
PO Box 38
Crowborough
Sussex TW6 2YP

Vibes
Mrs D. Frankish M Rad A
4 Relton Terrace
Monkseaton
Whitley Bay
Tyne & Wear NE25 8DY
Radionic homoeopathic remedies for ME, candida and
stopping smoking.

Labscan
Biomedical Screening Service
Silver Birches
Private Road
Rodborough Common
Stroud
Gloucestershire GL5 5BT
Tel 01435 873446/873668   Fax 01435 878588
An independent laboratory established to provide a non-
invasive simple-to-use comprehensive diagnostic service
for nutritionists and other practitioners who wish to
determine the ecological status of their patients intestinal
tract.

Federation of Aromatherapists
46 Dalkeith Road
London SE21

Nutrition Associates
Galtres House
Lysander Close
Clifton Moorgate
York YO3 0XB
Medical practice: candida/allergy testing, nutritional profiles, full spectrum lighting.

Cirrus Associates
Food and Environmental Consultancy
Little Hintock
Kington Magna
Gillingham
Dorset SP8 5EW
Tel 01747 838165
A wide range of products including VDU screen protectors, allergy-safe kettles and cooking appliances. Advice on allergies and special diets.

Health Plus Ltd
PO Box 86
Seaford
East Sussex BN25 4ZW
Tel 01323 492096
Supplies of convenient Candida Control pack and other products.

General Index

145

symptoms 2, 4
systemic candidiasis 3–4

tea 19
treatment, self-help
   methods 1, 6–7

vegetable stock cubes 26
vegetable stock
   powder 26
vegetables 13–14
   combining 79

cooking methods 73
   raw 48–51
vitamin deficiency 3
vitamins 7, 11

weight loss 8–9, 51
wheat 15–16
   alternatives 15–16
wheat flour,
   alternatives 16
withdrawal symptoms 9

Index to Recipes